31 Days to Overcoming Insomnia
Unlock Deep Sleep Secrets

Effective Strategies for Restful Sleep and Lasting Renewal

Dr. Cheryl T. Williams
Dr. Emmanuel J. Williams I

© 2025 by Dr. Cheryl T. Williams, LMHC, CPM / Dr. Emmanuel J. Williams I

ISBN 979-8-9988221-1-7

All rights reserved. No portion of this book may be reproduced, stored in a retrieval system, or transmitted in any form or by any means—electronic, mechanical, photocopy, recording, scanning, or other—except for brief quotations in critical reviews or articles, without the prior written permission of the authors.

Scripture quotations marked (KJV) are taken from the KING JAMES VERSION, public domain. Scripture quotations marked (NIV) are taken from the Holy Bible, New International Version®, NIV®. Copyright © 1973, 1978, 1984, 2011 by Biblica, Inc.™ Used by permission of Zondervan. All rights reserved worldwide. www.zondervan.comThe "NIV" and "New International Version" are trademarks registered in the United States Patent and Trademark Office by Biblica, Inc.™ Scripture quotations are from the ESV® Bible (The Holy Bible, English Standard Version®), copyright© 2001 by Crossway Bibles, a publishing ministry of Good News Publishers. Used by permission. All rights reserved.

*A Guided Journal and Workbook for
Mental, Emotional, and Spiritual Renewal*

TABLE OF CONTENTS

Acknowledgments i
Disclosure ii
Introduction iii

Your Preparation for The Journey

Chapter 1 - Sleep Is an Act of Faith 1
Chapter 2 - Getting Into Position For 31 Days 5
Chapter 3 - Starting Your 31 Days 8

Your 31-Day Journal

Day 1 - The Power of Rest: Unlocking the Key to Sound Sleep 14
Day 2 - Covered By Grace: Trust God's Protection 20
Day 3 - Adjusting Your Mental Frequency 26
Day 4 - Digital Detox: Reclaiming Peace from Screens 33
Day 5 - Sleep & Mental Health: Rest for The Mind & Spirit 40
Day 6 - Insomnia Is from Hell: Breaking Free from Sleeplessness 47
Day 7 - God's Promise 54
Day 8 - Trusting God's Wisdom Over Your Own Understanding 60
Day 9 - Safeguarding Your Environment 66
Day 10 - Christ Provides You with The Strength You Need 74
Day 11 - Morning Mental Clarity 81
Day 12 - His Spirit Dwells in You 87
Day 13 - The Power That Operates Within You 94
Day 14 - Igniting Your Inner Spark: The Transformative Power of Self-Care 101
Day 15 - Keep Pushing: The Relentless Power of Perseverance 110
Day 16 - Your Mouth Will Speak Life 119
Day 17 - Dream It to Existence 126
Day 18 - Refreshing Rest 132
Day 19 - Surrender & Rest 138
Day 20 - Unwinding: Finding Peace in The Stillness 143
Day 21 - The Importance of Downtime for Mental Health 149
Day 22 - Be Connected to The Secret Place 156
Day 23 - Sleep-Friendly Foods: What to Eat for Better Zzzs 162

Day 24 - From Pain to Peace: Navigating Sleep After Trauma 169
Day 25 - Forgive Yourself & Sleep 176
Day 26 - The Word in Action: Bringing Scripture to Life 182
Day 27 - Not Today, Devil: Claiming Victory Over Your Sleep 188
Day 28 - Beyond The 31 Nights: A Lasting Commitment to Rest 194
Day 29 - Restoring Peace: Letting Go of Grudges Before Bed 200
Day 30 - Embracing Forgiveness 207
Day 31 - Silent Mind, Restful Sleep – Navigating Your Subconscious 214
Conclusion – Moving Forward in Continuous Sound Sleep and Rejuvenation 222
Resources

ACKNOWLEDGEMENTS

Sleep is more than rest—it is a consecrated pause,
a divine invitation to trust, release, and be restored.

This journal was born from a deep passion to help others regain their peace, nightly, through deliberate reflection and spiritual restoration.

To my co-writer, Emmanuel—thank you for your unwavering faith, shared vision, and constant dedication throughout this journey. Your insight, creativity, and commitment have brought depth and resonance to these pages, and I am deeply grateful to walk this path with you.

To our editor, Anjeanette Alexander—your expertise, discernment, and thoughtful feedback have been invaluable. Your ability to polish ideas while honoring the heart behind them has not only refined this work but lifted it. Thank you for your endurance, accuracy, and belief in the message.

We extend our sincere gratitude to Kingdom News Today for their exceptional layout and cover design work on this journal. Your professional creativity and dedication transformed this project into an experience that exceeded what we originally expected. Your peaceful and polished presentation gives readers an enhanced experience while perfectly capturing the essence of our journal.

To those who encouraged and supported me along the way—family, friends, and mentors—your prayers, words of confirmation, and presence have supported me. Each step of this process has been enriched by your encouragement.

To our readers—this journal is for you. May each page invite you to slow down, lean in, and embrace the kind of rest that reaches beyond the physical. May you discover, in stillness, the profound peace that transcends understanding.

And above all, to God, the source of perfect peace—we dedicate this work.
May it serve as a container of healing, rebuilding, and transformation for every heart that seeks rest.

With deep gratitude,
Cheryl & Emmanuel

DISCLAIMER

This journal functions as a space for personal reflection and spiritual encouragement while providing general wellness support. Even though the author holds credentials as both a Licensed Mental Health Counselor and a Certified Christian Counselor, this journal cannot replace professional counseling services or medical treatment for mental health needs.

This journal does not create a counselor-client relationship between its author and its readers. The content serves only to provide information and inspiration: therefore, it must not be used as a diagnosis or treatment method.

Seek professional support from a licensed healthcare provider if you have ongoing sleep problems or mental health issues or find yourself in an emergency situation.

Reading this journal is completely optional, and the author takes no responsibility for any results that stem from its use.

INTRODUCTION

Are you tired of battling the night — and losing?
Are you lying awake with your mind racing, your body restless, and sleep feeling like a distant dream? You're not alone. Insomnia — the unwelcome companion — disrupts our rest, drains our strength, and seeps into our emotions, minds, and bodies. The burden is overwhelming, but the answer lies deeper than you might think.

What if the solution isn't just habit control, but a transformation of your entire approach to rest — body, mind, and soul? Imagine rediscovering authentic, restorative sleep by addressing the root of your insomnia and inviting peace into every part of your life.

Welcome to a 31-day journey that will help you do just that. This isn't another sleep aid or quick fix. It's a whole-person, therapeutic guide to reclaiming your rest. Through practical strategies, **Rest Renewal Coaching**, and heartfelt reflections, you'll not only sleep — you'll heal.

Each day, you'll engage in a powerful and intentional blend of:

- **Cognitive Renewal Statements** to reframe your mind and reset your beliefs about rest.
- **Guided Reflections** to invite deep insight into what's truly keeping you awake.
- **Mindful Rest Practices** that gently transform your habits and renew your body.
- **Rest Renewal Coaching** — bite-sized encouragement to strengthen your resilience and promote deeper calm.
- **Evening Reflections** to close your day with clarity and peace.

These daily rhythms — with their morning and evening cognitive renewal statements, guided reflections, mindful rest practices, and thoughtful evening reflections — are designed to quiet your mind, restore your body, and help you reclaim deep, healing rest.

Through this journey, you'll realize sleeping well isn't just about falling asleep — it's about living a life of restfulness where your heart, mind, and body find renewal. It's creating a rhythm where, when your head touches the pillow, stress falls away and peace takes its place.

Over the next 31 days, you'll uncover the hidden patterns behind your sleepless nights and build new rhythms of mindful, restorative rest. With daily practice and reflection, you'll not only prevent insomnia — you'll discover joy, balance, and rejuvenation as essential parts of your life.

This isn't just about surviving the night — it's about waking up each morning with fresh strength, clear purpose, and unshakable calm.

So, are you ready to finally rest — fully, deeply, and fearlessly?

Let's take back sleep and live again in harmony, vitality, and strength.

Welcome to your transformation. These 31 days could change everything.

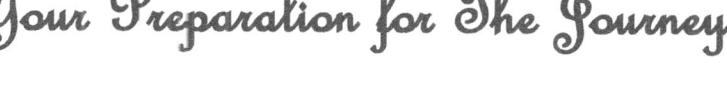
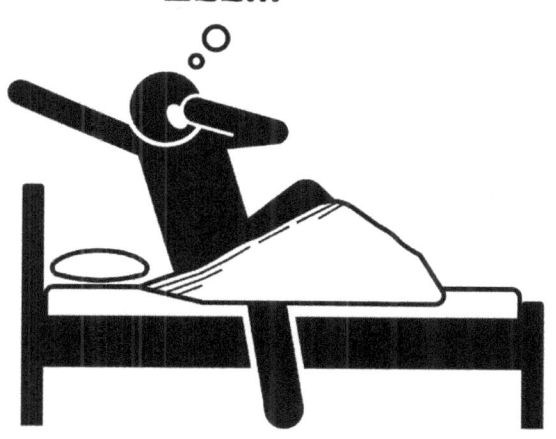

Chapter 1
SLEEP IS AN ACT OF FAITH

Rest is a demonstration of faith in God.

Sleep shows trust.
The act of sleeping is an act of faith.
Resting is surrendering.

Sweet sleep is a demonstration of faith in God.

Introduction
Sleep is one of the basic foundations of human life, and yet a lot of people lose a lot of sleep most nights. The culprit for sleepless nights includes tireless worrying, anxiety, and stress—which is the reason why there are no manuals written to address the silent half of the nights when sleep eludes us. Sleeplessness occurs more often than one can imagine. From a biblical perspective, sleep is not just a physiological and functional necessity, but also an act of trust. When we sleep, we relinquish control, which is an act of faith in our Lord Jesus Christ, trusting and believing that He is faithful to take care of us as we peacefully rest. In this chapter, we will discuss six key godly concepts that will serve as the biblical basis for sleep as a demonstration of trust in God and how the contentment of trusting God's provision and God's protection will lead to restorative and peaceful rest.

1. Relying on Divine Protection
Psalms 4:8 (NIV) is a portion of scripture that explicitly links sleep with trust in God:
"In peace I will lie down and sleep, for you alone, LORD, make me dwell in safety."

The psalmist claims – rest is what You give me, Lord, and it is You alone my soul is convinced of. In You, Lord, I trust; let me never be ashamed. Here, he enjoys the kind of security that arises from knowing that, with God on his side, his life is in safe hands, and we can be assured of the same promise. In ancient times, as now, sleeping is a vulnerable state—in that state, we are unconscious, oblivious of what's happening in our immediate surroundings and totally defenseless. The psalmist was sleeping at ease because he knew the Lord was watching over him. This suggests that sound sleep is inextricably linked to knowledge of the Most High's willingness to care for and protect us. Hence, sleep is more than just attaining physical rest, but a profound spiritual act of surrendering and trust.

31 Days to Overcoming Insomnia

Despite all our weariness and misery, God still remains our Father—awake when we are not, with a care that has never wavered, eyes unwavering, yes, we will trust. If we could come to experience sleep in this way, then it would give us a new sense of freedom as we settled down each night. Therefore, the solution is not to force ourselves to sleep, but to let it occur naturally on its own. If God holds the world in His hands, certainly He has you in His hands. Go get your Zzzzs.

2. Reliance on Divine Provision

In **Matthew 6:25, 34 (KJV)**, Jesus speaks to His followers about the stresses of life:

> *"Therefore, I say unto you, take no thought for your life, what ye shall eat, or what ye shall drink; nor yet for your body, what ye shall put on. Is not life more than meat, and the body than raiment? Take therefore no thought for the morrow: for the morrow shall take thought for the things of itself. Sufficient unto the day is the evil thereof."*

The lesson here is simple: trusting in God's provision can lead to feeling at rest, while worry erodes trust in God and can lead to restlessness. So many sleepless nights are the result of worrying about one's inadequate resources and opportunities in the future. Jesus calls us to lay aside our anxieties and bring our needs to Him, to seek God's kingdom first, and to trust that God will provide for us.

When we accept this reality, every night can become an opportunity to go to bed at peace, trusting in God's sovereignty over all things. In turning off the lights and entrusting ourselves to sleep, we trust that God will be our Provider, because He already is.

3. Trusting in God's Sovereignty Over Circumstances

A major cause of sleep deprivation is the need to be in control of every circumstance. If life seems uncertain and perplexing, don't feel obligated to take charge and sort through every detail. Most times, things work out on their own. Additionally, the good news of the Bible reminds us that God is sovereign over all things, so we don't have to be in control of everything.

In **Proverbs 3:5-6 (NIV)**, we are instructed: *"Trust in the Lord with all your heart and lean not on your own understanding; in all your ways submit to him, and he will make your paths straight."*

The lesson here is that peace is found in trusting God's leadership and sovereignty. We should not carry the burdens of the world nor should we expect to know everything either. Instead, we are to trust God's leading so that our souls are liberated from cumbersome burdens and sleep will come easily when God's perfect wisdom directs our paths despite the unknown.

4. Relying on God's Care During Tough Times
The Bible doesn't deny that life can be tumultuous, but it does promise that God will be with us in the struggle. In **Psalm 121:3-4 (NIV)**, we read: *"He will not let your foot slip—he who watches over you will not slumber; indeed, he who watches over Israel will neither slumber nor sleep."*

These verses show a comforting image of God as the vigilant guardian, patiently staying awake to protect those who are weighed down with life's ever-present burdens. When we face times that are full of trials, finding rest can often be elusive, as tumultuous thoughts cycle through a myriad of resolutions to a problem. A busy mind makes it impossible to be still, which precedes a good night's rest. This portion of scripture, however, should bring some comfort to our soul. It reassures us that God "does not slumber nor sleep." Therefore, since God is awake, we can go to sleep knowing God is at work —even in the darkest of nights.

5. The Sabbath Rest: A Sign of Trust
The Sabbath rest became a refrain throughout Scripture. The Sabbath required the Israelites to pull away from work, put down their burdens, and put their trust in God. In Exodus 20:8-10, on the seventh day, the Israelites were commanded to refrain from work one day each week to show their trust in God's promise that six days of labor would be enough to sustain them. To observe the Sabbath day is a way of showing that they believed God would take care of them even though they were not working.

The practice of Sabbath rest can be adopted as it relates to sleep. Each night when we go to sleep, we leave behind whatever we aimed to accomplish and entrust ourselves to God to continue providing for our needs. We put our trust in God while we sleep, just as the Israelites did on the Sabbath, because we know that He is at work.

6. The Example of Trust and Rest Exemplified by Jesus
Even Jesus sometimes trusts God enough to fall asleep. In Mark 4:38-39, Jesus is sleeping in a boat with His disciples when there is a storm. When they draw His attention to the situation yelling: 'Teacher, don't you care if we drown?" He wakes up and responds to the thunderstorm with "Peace! Be still!" Then He turns to His disciples and asks: "Why are you so afraid? Have you still no faith in God?"

Jesus was able to sleep in the storm because He trusted totally in the Father's care for Him. Jesus' life and mission were safely held in God's hands, and so He had nothing to fear. The lesson here is that we, too, can face the raging fury of life and storms in the knowledge that we are protected and that God is ultimately in control of our lives and our missions.

There is Blessed Assurance When You Rest in God

In the end, the act of sleep is a way of showing one's daily reliance on God. Anytime we lay down to rest, we are admitting that we are not in charge—God is. We rely on Him to sustain us, to heal us, and to direct us through the storms of life. Through this trust, we release fear that otherwise impedes our sleep.

In Scripture, rest and sweet sleep are guaranteed to those who trust the Lord. As we mature spiritually and our faith grows, may it be revealed to us by the Holy Ghost that getting good rest is not just a physical necessity, but a spiritual act. A spiritual act of surrender to the Most-High God who neither slumbers nor sleeps and who securely holds our lives in the palm of His hands.

Chapter 2
GETTING INTO POSITION FOR 31 DAYS

Welcome to the 31-day challenge for beating insomnia and getting the restful sleep you've always deserved. Before we get into the tactics, practices, and tips that will lead you through the next several weeks, it is critical that you "get in position."

What does it look like to "get in position" for this journey? It's not only about priming your brain for transformation. It's about putting yourself in the right place spiritually, emotionally, and physically to be ready for the change. By prepping in these four areas, you'll not only be prepared for it, but more importantly, you'll have peace and purpose on your side for the next 31 days.

1. Positioning Your Mind: Letting Go of Old Beliefs

When insomnia strikes, the first thing to get rid of is the psychological impediment. After having sleeplessness for a long time, it is very easy to get stuck in a mindset of "that's how sleeplessness works" or that it will always be a struggle. But to really get it right, you have to set your brain up for possibilities.

Scriptural Wisdom
"Do not conform to this world but be transformed by the renewing of your mind." – Romans 12:2 (NIV)

Guided Reflections
Ask yourself if there are any assumptions you have that limit your sleep? Are you afraid you will never sleep well again? Is it too late to make a shift? Just sit and jot them down and remember that these thoughts aren't true; they're just not last minute, and they can be changed if you work hard.

Mindful Rest Practices
Before beginning this process, compose a letter to yourself as if it were addressed to a friend. In it, acknowledge the struggles you've faced, but also remind yourself that you are worthy of tranquility, peace, and restoration. Reaffirm that your past sleep patterns don't define your future, and that change is possible.

Prayer
Dear God, I hand over to You my sleep worries, my sleep fears, and my doubts. Let me have a sense that things are changeable and allow me to refocus my mind in

order to believe in Your power to restore my mind to calm and rest. I lay my fears in Your palms and ask You for a remedy.

2. Positioning Your Heart: Opening Up to Healing and Peace

Before authentic healing can take place, you need to position your heart to receive the peace that God offers. Insomnia often stems from deeper emotional struggles—stress, anxiety, grief, or unresolved trauma. These feelings can block the peaceful rest that you long for. As you start this journey, it's important to be open to addressing these emotions and inviting God's healing presence into your life.

Scriptural Wisdom
"Come to Me, all you who are weary and burdened, and I will give you rest." – Matthew 11:28 (NIV)

Guided Reflections
Consider for a moment the emotional origins of your sleeplessness. What concerns or concerns get you up at night? Have you had hurts in the past or stress that you are overwhelmed by today? Write it in your journal and ask God to quiet those parts of your heart.

Mindful Rest Practices
Work on clearing your mind at bedtime. Every night, take a few minutes to note any stress or anxiety. And then with every deep breath, lay them out one by one into God's hands. You can even perform this exercise at the same time every night to develop a ritual of submission before going to bed.

Prayer
Dear God, I bring my struggles to Thee. Heal my heart bleeds, soothe my panicked mind, and calm me down. Help me to learn how to let You carry my load for me and that You are doing all things for me when I am asleep. I pray Your peace is in my heart and mind.

3. Positioning Your Body: Creating a Restful Space and Routine

The environment and circadian rhythms of your body significantly affect the quality of your sleep. To prepare for sleep, you need to prepare your surroundings and physical habits for rest. This involves creating a sleep-friendly environment and practicing bodily movements that signal to your body that it's time to rest.

Scriptural Wisdom
"He leads me to lie down in lush meadows; He takes me to still waters." – Psalm 23:2 (NIV)

Unlock Deep Sleep Secrets

Guided Reflections
Examine your current sleep environment. Is your bedroom serene, relaxing, and peaceful? Do you have bedtime routines that help you relax? Write about what you can do to enhance your room, whether it's turning off the lights, keeping the room quiet, or clearing the space.

Mindful Rest Practices
Be determined to make your bedroom a relaxing place to sleep. First, remove any distractions—unplug gadgets, dim lights, and add comforters, such as blankets, soothing music, or scented candles. Also, be mindful of your bedtime routine: make it a point to begin cooling off at least 30 minutes before bed.

Prayer
Dear God, I want to live in a meditative state that's soothing to my mind, body, and soul. Teach me to know how to make adjustments in my daily schedule and in my body to appreciate the rest that You have placed in me. Let me sleep securely and safely with You.

4. Positioning Your Spirit: Trusting in God's Provision for Rest
The final bit of putting yourself in gear is setting your soul up to surrender and rest and be restored in Him. If you're an insomniac, you might not notice how God has a plan for everything, including your sleep. It's a spiritual rebirth as much as a physical and emotional purification.

Scripture Wisdom
"In peace I will lie down and sleep, for You alone, Lord, make me dwell in safety." – Psalm 4:8 (NIV)

Guided Reflections
Which of your spiritual dimensions do you need to focus on in order to be at peace? Have you completely given God your sleep needs, or are you in control where you should be? Ask yourself where you can put God in your healing rest.

Mindful Rest Practices
Each night, spend just a few minutes before bed inviting God into your sleep time. Say a mantra or scripture, such as Psalm 4:8, that you will be provided for by God while you sleep. Repeat this affirmation over and over as you hold your breath, a prayer to open your heart to sleep in confidence.

Prayer
Dear God, You know rest is what You made my body, my mind, and my soul to be. Help me give up my control and let peace surround me. You will quiet me so that I can sleep knowing that You are always with me.

Chapter 3
STARTING YOUR 31 DAYS

Congratulations on taking the first steps to eliminating insomnia and getting back the sleep your body, brain, and soul sorely craves! This 31-day journey will take you through a process of change, one that will provide you with the resources to end the nightly cycle once and for all. With hands-on advice, reflective prompts, exercises, scripture, and prayer, you're not merely trying to drift off, you're looking for whole-body rejuvenation.

This chapter is about beginning—that's how you get started for the next 31 days, getting your heart, brain, and body ready for transformation, and knowing that it will happen through consistency. Even if it isn't at times, easy or fast going, remember that better sleep and renewal are not a sprint. By consciously working on it, putting your trust in it and continuing, you will see change in your sleep habits and above all in your health.

1. Starting with a Heart of Hope: Setting Your Intention for This Journey

Before we get to the actual action steps for the next 31 days, you need to get focused on the endgame. This is not a 31-day program; it is a way to reset your relationship with sleep, your emotional wellness, and your spiritual well-being. To fight insomnia, you will have to delve not only into the physiological aspects of sleep, but the emotional and spiritual as well. If you start with a heart of hope, then you'll have the strength to endure the days to come.

Scripture Wisdom
"I can do all things by Christ who strengthens me." – Philippians 4:13 (NIV)

Guided Reflections
Ask yourself what your sleep challenges are right now and how they affect your life. Write down how physically, emotionally, and spiritually affected you have been by these obstacles. Here's an invitation to bring hope into the picture. How do you think you can get things to shift? How would you feel if you got rest and refreshment from sleeplessness?

Mindful Rest Practices
Breathe and let go of your worries. Write a surrender prayer for your sleep problems, telling God that you're ready for recovery. Here is where you begin: a break with the past and a focus on the promise of the future.

Unlock Deep Sleep Secrets

Prayer
'My heart is teeming with promise,' I cry to You. I know You are right here with me. Remind me to rest in Your promises and to relinquish my anxiety to You. And I know that You are leading me to sleep and recovery. Give me the strength to endure this and see it out.

2. Assessing Your Current Sleep Habits: Understanding Where You Are

To move forward, it's important to first recognize where you are. Over the next few days, you'll take a close look at your current sleep patterns, identifying the habits and routines that may be contributing to your insomnia. By assessing your current situation, you'll be able to make informed, strategic changes in the days ahead.

Scripture Wisdom
"But let each one examine his own work, and then he will have rejoicing in himself alone, and not in another." – Galatians 6:4 (NIV)

Guided Reflections
Take a moment to check in on how you're sleeping. What is your usual nighttime routine? Where are you when you go to sleep and when you wake up? Note any habits that come to mind such as things that can cause you to not sleep, like screen time, stress, or waking up during an uncoordinated time.

Mindful Rest Practices
For the next three nights, write a simple sleep diary. Track the following:

- The time you went to bed
- The time you woke up
- Any interruptions to your sleep (waking up in the middle of the night, difficulty falling asleep)
- Any activities or thoughts before bed (screen use, stress levels, emotional state)

After three days, review your sleep journal and note any patterns or habits that may need to be addressed.

Prayer
Dear God, show me the behaviors and routines that are blocking my sleep. Please help me see where I can change and give me the judgment and strength to do so. I am asking You to lead me through these small but powerful acts of making it sleep again.

31 Days to Overcoming Insomnia

3. Establishing Your Sleep Goals: Setting a Vision for Change

In the first day of this 31-day program, you should make concrete, doable objectives for yourself. What does good sleep look like to you? Is it going to sleep quicker, staying asleep all night or waking up feeling absolutely fresh. By establishing your goals, you will have a clear vision of what you are working toward. These goals will serve as your motivation during days when the process feels difficult.

Scripture Wisdom
"Write the vision and make it plain on tablets, that he may run who reads it." – Habakkuk 2:2 (NIV)

Guided Reflections
Spend some time visualizing your dream sleep. What would it be like to get up feeling better? What would you do to ensure your sleep was therapeutic and healing? Make a list of your 31-day resolutions — whether it's getting to sleep earlier, sleeping better, or waking less at night.

Mindful Rest Practices
Note down your sleep goals, something personal and inspiring. Make this list somewhere that you can see, like a journal, or a wall, or a mirror, so you can remind yourself daily what you are working toward. Throughout these exercises in this journal, think back to these objectives and see where you are coming along.

Prayer
Dear God, I am bringing my sleep goals to You today. Allow me to see how my need for rest is in Your plan for my life. Please give me the power and perseverance to stay on track with these objectives and the grace to know that progress will be at Your time. May it bring me more tranquility and recovery in You.

4. Making Your Sleep A Habit: A Way to Stick to It

Once you are on the 31-day kick, it is essential that you build consistency in your habits. This includes having a sleep routine at night that tells your body that it's time to relax and go to sleep. Developing a quiet practice will get your mind and body used to calming down and getting into sleep mode.

Scripture Wisdom
"The Lord will preserve your going out and your coming in from this day forth and the age to come." – Psalm 121:8

Guided Reflections
What do you do to chill out and wind down at night? Does any ritual make you feel relaxed and at peace: like reading, writing, praying? Think of calming tasks you can do every night.

Unlock Deep Sleep Secrets

Mindful Rest Practices
Develop a consistent sleep routine that works for you. Consider activities such as:

Leaving the lights on 30 minutes before going to bed.
Limiting screen time.
Reading scripture or a devotional.
Writing in your journal.
Deep breathing or some relaxation practice.

Prayer
Dear God, I want to thank you for the wisdom to embrace rest as a gift and the discipline to make it a regular part of my life. Help me build a calm routine, where I can embrace every night and look forward to better health and clarity.

May my sleep be a mirror image of stability and well-being, and may I honor my body as a temple through rest. In Your name, I pray. Amen.

Your First Step Toward Renewal
When you are starting out, remember it's not going to be overnight, but it will come with consistent effort and hard work. Some days might be hard and even discouraged, but you should understand that every day is a win. Be willing, be dependent on the methods and insights you're building up, and count on the power of God to get you through.

When you begin with intention, take inventory of where you are, make sure you have targets, and have regular rest routines in place, you are creating the foundation for rest and healing. Keep the hope and grit going. And you are not the only one doing this. God is with you, and He will draw nigh to you at night for a peace.

You're not merely trying to sleep better; you're making a whole new you that will make you rest, reset, and re-energized. Let's get started, one day at a time, night after night.

Your 31-Day Journal

Day 1
THE POWER OF REST: UNLOCKING THE KEY TO SOUND SLEEP

Philippians 4:6-7 (NIV):
"Do not be anxious about anything, but in every situation, by prayer and petition, with thanksgiving, present your requests to God. And the peace of God, which transcends all understanding, will guard your hearts and your minds in Christ Jesus."

We're all hard-working people yet rest rarely comes to us. We race through life, eyes locked on endless to-do lists, fingers snapping from one task to the next. We believe that doing more will give us more. But the truth is sobering we are slowly killing ourselves—one by one—by denying our bodies and minds the very thing they've been longing for all along: sleep.

Rest is a high art in a world that glorifies exhaustion. We are told to stay up later, work longer, hustle harder, and sleep less—as if busyness is the badge of honor. But here's the truth: without rest, there is no life. Rest isn't weakness; it's the hidden strength that shapes our bodies, sharpens our minds, and steadies our hearts. And the beauty of rest is not found only in the hours we sleep, but in the intentional pauses we carve out—moments where we stop, breathe, and allow God's peace to reset our souls.

And yet so few of us even get a good night's sleep. It is the nights when we lie in bed, a bloated wreck, and our brains are alive and well: beat with tension, jammed with worries, swirling with thoughts. We don't sleep and we wake up the next morning drained.

But what if sleep were the secret to…not sleep but life? If sleep could alter our sleep… our life!

Unlock Deep Sleep Secrets

The Healing Force of Sleep: A Divine Call to Arms

Philippians 4:6–7 invites us into deeper rest. This moving scripture reminds us that true repose is not found in the absence of problems but in the presence of God's peace. And this peace is unlike anything the world can offer—it is an incomprehensible calm that flows from surrender. When we release our anxieties into God's hands, He places a divine guard over our hearts and minds, shielding us from the chaos and disturbances that steal our rest.

Listen! Rest is not just about getting enough hours of sleep. Real rest begins when our hearts find a safe dwelling place in God—free from fear, worry, and anxiety. Sleep becomes more than physical renewal; it becomes sacred space, the room we create when we let go and enter the stillness of God. It is in this stillness that true rest is born.

Sleep And Anxiety: The Connection Between Them Both?

Anxiety is one of the most serious roadblocks to rest. It gets our brains all warped, unfocused, and disconnected from the silence we need to fall asleep. You know what it's like, sitting in bed, exhausted, but unable to put your head down. The thought of never-ending tasks, never-answered issues, and the unknowable about the future race through your head, and they will not allow you to rest. The body is maybe tired, but the brain keeps ticking over and you are out of it.

And Philippians 4:6-7 provides the antidote: *"Be not anxious about anything."* An easy thing to say, but one that can feel incomprehensible when fear takes over. But here's the thing: anxiety is an option. Thoughts do go through our heads sometimes; we do manage our reaction to them. It tells us to surrender the fear in prayer and petition—to turn our anxieties over to God and allow Him to take control.

We stop holding the burden of our anxieties, and then peace comes in. When we relinquish, rest is available. The more we put our confidence in God's power to take care of us, the better off we can be. It is not a lack of noise, this quiet; it is the presence of something bigger. That's the calm when we believe in something greater than our worries, the calm to go to sleep.

The Power of Surrender

Rest begins with surrender. It demands that we abandon the will to 'run' things, to forfeit the ever-present wish to prepare, repair, or settle them all. Rest requires trust. And we have to believe that even in this state of doubt, we're not alone. God is at work, even if we don't see all of it.

If we leave all our worries in God's hands, we allow sleep in. It is not something passive. It's a deliberate decision to not move, to not be in charge, to simply be. And there is calm, that silence.

31 Days to Overcoming Insomnia

This evening, before going to bed, think of the power of surrender. Be sure to clear away all the thoughts and fears that are keeping you up at night before getting into bed. Speak them into the hand of God in prayer. Seek Him, for His stillness, for His promise to guard your heart and mind. And you do so by unlocking the key to deep sleep. And you are asking God's tranquility to guard your mind and your body, and to live more fully.

The Transformational Power of Rest

And once we start recognizing the real magic of sleep, we realize that it is not only about a good night's rest, but also about a life lived in peace and trust. Rest doesn't happen in bed; it's the way we go about our days. It comes when we give up our fears, surrender to God's sovereign will, and let go of the need for perfection.

And this rest is different when we practice it. We fall asleep better because our brains are in harmony. We come up refreshed because we've given our bodies a chance to repair and recharge. We pass through life in less confusion and with less anxiety because we've mastered surrender.

What if you could live a life in which you no longer have to carry worry in your mind, where your mind was not consumed by the madness of the world? What if you could wake up every morning feeling at ease knowing that whatever happens you are not alone? This is the force of rest, the stillness beyond knowledge, the stillness that clings to your heart and your head.

Rest is Your Birthright

Rest is not a luxury. It is your right, a right given to you by your Creator. And once you tap into the secret of sleep, you tap into the serenity that will change everything.

Philippians 4:6-7 invites you to that tranquility and asks you to let go of your worries, forsake all your anxieties and concerns, and let God take care of you. When you allow this harmony into your life, you will not only get better sleep, but you will also feel better overall.

So before you fall asleep tonight, take note of this: Rest is a choice. Peace is within your reach. So, give up your worries, let go of controlling thoughts, and let the peace of God keep watch over your heart and your mind. And there in that quiet, you'll get the restful night you've been craving.

Prayer for the Journey

Dear God and my Lord Jesus, my High Priest who is touched with every feeling of my infirmity (insomnia, unnecessary sleeplessness), before I go to bed tonight, I place all my anxieties and cares at Your feet. I trust in Your care to experience sweet sleep tonight. Your word commands me not to worry about anything, and so I trust in You and in the power of Your might. I'm so grateful for what You've done for me and it's in that attitude of

Unlock Deep Sleep Secrets

gratitude that I voice this need and problem to You. Thank you for Your blessings in my life, the mercies You've extended to me and Your steadfast love that never ceases. You commanded me to be careful for nothing, so I declare, I am careful for nothing. I am not going to let the issues in my mind pull me in different directions. Right now, I receive Your peace, the peace that surpasses all understanding. I welcome the sweet sleep You promised because Your peace is able to guard my mind like a sentinel. I decree to sweet sleep that you are free to flood my body, soul, and spirit right now in Jesus' name. Amen.

As you pray the prayer of Philippians 4:6-7, you are demonstrating a deep trust in God's nurturing presence, paving the way for restful sleep while embracing the comforting assurance of a peace that transcends all understanding.

31 Days to Overcoming Insomnia

JOURNAL
"Sound Sleep is Important"

Morning Cognitive Renewal Statement

- I release my anxieties into God's hands. I trust that His peace will fill my heart and mind, allowing me to rest deeply and peacefully.

Morning Journal Guided Reflections

Set Intentions: What intentions can I set today to manage my anxiety? How can I focus on gratitude rather than worry?

_____
_____
_____

Identify Worries: What specific anxieties or worries am I facing today? How can I present them to God?

_____
_____
_____

Positive Visualization: Visualize a peaceful day ahead. What does it look like? How can I embrace peace in my interactions?

_____
_____
_____

Evening Cognitive Renewal Statements

- I appreciate the ability to rest, and I'm confident my sleep will revive my mind and body. I believe that my sleep will restore everything that is broken.

Evening Journal Guided Reflections

Gratitude Reflection: What are three things I am grateful for today? How did they help ease my anxiety?

_____
_____
_____

Unlock Deep Sleep Secrets

Releasing Worries: List the worries that occupied my mind today. How did I surrender them to God and trust in His peace?

_____
_____
_____
_____

Peaceful Moments: Reflect on moments during the day when I felt calm. What contributed to those feelings, and how can I cultivate more of them?

_____
_____
_____
_____

Mindful Rest Practices

- **Prayer and Reflection:** Spend a few minutes in prayer, lifting your anxieties to God. Use the time to express your worries and ask for peace. Consider journaling about the experience afterward.

- **Mindful Breathing:** Practice deep breathing exercises for 5-10 minutes. Inhale deeply through your nose, hold for a moment, and exhale slowly through your mouth. Visualize your breath carrying away anxiety and filling you with peace.

- **Journaling Exercise:** Dedicate a section of your journal to "Dear Anxiety." Write letters addressing your fears and worries, acknowledging them, and then respond to them with affirmations and prayers.

- **Gratitude Journaling:** Each evening, write down at least three things you're grateful for. Reflect on how gratitude can shift your focus away from anxiety.

- **Meditation on Scripture:** Spend time meditating on Philippians 4:6-7. Write down any insights or feelings that arise. Consider how this scripture can guide you in managing anxiety.

- **Relaxing Bedtime Routine:** Create a calming bedtime routine that includes reading, gentle stretching, or listening to soothing music. Allow this time to signal to your mind and body that it's time to rest.

Day 2
COVERED BY GRACE: TRUSTING GOD'S PROTECTION

Psalm 4:8 (ESV):
*"In peace I will both lie down and sleep;
for you alone, O Lord, make me dwell in safety."*

Imagine lying in bed at night while the world around you feel noisy, unsettled, and disorganized—yet you are perfectly at peace. Your body is still, your mind is quiet, and deep inside you know, all is well. You're not simply drifting into sleep; you're resting in the embrace of the supreme Defender—God Himself. His arms cover you; His presence shields you, and not even fear dares to disturb your rest.

And that's the promise of Psalm 4:8: "In peace I will lie down and sleep, for You alone, Lord, make me dwell in safety."

But what if you could have this deep stillness all night? What if every night's slumber was an act of trust—an expression of your faith in God's protection?

We live in a world constantly on edge, where threats, real and imagined—appear around every corner. For many, sleep feels like a battle. We have our heads flitting with unwelcome thoughts and our hearts pound, burdened by the weight we cannot control.
Yet in Psalm 4:8, God has a plan for us. He does not simply say you can sleep; God declares that you will sleep -in safety and in peace. It's the reassurance that, no matter the storms around you, God Himself cradles you in His grace, guards you with His love, and shelters you under His unfailing protection.

Unlock Deep Sleep Secrets

The Grace of His Protection

Everybody fears the unknowns. Anxiety rises when we feel insecure or uncertain about what lies ahead. Whether it's a physical threat, financial challenges, marital tension or another hidden worry, our minds buzz "what ifs" that rob us of peace and keep rest far away. If we were to place our faith in God's protection, it might be a lofty dream, but God's protection isn't just a pipedream—it's an active, real-time protective shield that covers us night and day.

God's shield is not a distant, involuntary operation. It is not a dream or a distant hope. His protection is a living, active shield that surrounds us—moment by moment, day and night. His shield is not distant or impersonal. It is the grace of God at work. Grace that calms us in the middle of life's storms. Grace that guards our hearts when fear whispers its lies. Grace that allows us to sit in quiet confidence, knowing the One who holds the universe also holds us.

This grace is like a warm covering—wrapping around us, reminding us that we are never alone. When we trust God's protection, we are declaring that His mercy covers every place we walk and every fear we face.

Even in the darkest hours of the night, when fear feels the loudest, God's grace speaks louder still. His presence pours over us, not to frighten us, but to steady us. We are safe, cradled in His grace, guarded by His love, and sheltered under His unfailing protection.

Letting Go of Fear

Fear is one of the biggest stumbling blocks to good sleep. Fear is a thief—it steals our serenity, our joy, and the rest our bodies and minds so desperately need. Whether it's fear of the unknown or fear of harm, it often creeps into our hearts at night when the day is done and our minds are no longer distracted.

But fear and peace cannot coexist. The more we surrender our anxieties to God, the more we experience the peace promised in Psalm 4:8: "In peace I will lie down and sleep, for you alone, Lord, make me dwell in safety." This peace is possible only because we trust in God's protective love. When we remember that He has already conquered fear, we can rest in the assurance that we are safe under His care.

That is the secret to overcoming fear and anxiety—not that we must control detail, but that God already holds all control. His shield does not stop protecting our bodies; it also guards our hearts, our minds, and our souls. When we release control and depend fully on Him, true rest becomes not just possible but promised.

31 Days to Overcoming Insomnia

God's Defender: A Shield for the Night

There is something powerful about God's protection at night. Darkness has a way of exposing our weakness. Our bodies may rest, but our minds often refuse. We let our brains whirl around and do the impossible, rewind, and repeat the mistakes of the past or project terror into the future. In those quiet hours, we can feel most defenseless, weighed down by what we cannot change or control.

But when we place our confidence in God's faithfulness, the night has no power over us. Psalm 4:8 assures us that the Lord keeps us "dwelling in safety." His protection is not a single event—it is an unending promise we can believe day and night. While we sleep and are at our most vulnerable, God is still our Savior, standing guard over us. His mercy never ends; when the sun sets and our eyes close, His everlasting arms surround us, covering us with peace and defending us with love.

Covering by Grace, Sleeping in His Care

The very name of God is beautiful: He is plentiful in grace. Grace is His loving kindness poured freely, unearned, underserved, yet always available. It's the cover we wear, the silence beyond knowledge, and the constant reminder that we are never alone.

When we remember that God wraps us in His love, we can close our eyes at night with complete confidence that we are safe in His arms. It doesn't mean life won't be hard or we won't have struggles. But it does mean that, no matter what comes, we are never abandoned.

To rest in God's care is to rest in His love. It is to lie down each night knowing that the Lord is present, providing for us, and shielding us from harm. His grace embraces us, and within that covering, we find the deep, soul-rest our hearts have been yearning for.

Prayer for the Journey

Dear God, You've been my shelter and the one in whom I experience true tranquility. As I make preparations for a restful sleep tonight, I decree that my mind is free from worry, fear, and all false alarms. Psalms 4:8 shows us that regardless of David's troubles and challenges, he was still able to lay himself down in peace and get sweet sleep because he had the assurance of Your favor. In like manner, I will lay myself down in peace and safety because of Your faithfulness to protect me. Though it may seem I am alone, yet I am not alone, for God is with me. Though it may seem that I have no guards to assist me, I decree the word of our Lord stands as a sentinel at the door of my mind. It is sufficient to protect me from sleep-disturbing thoughts. You are the only one who can truly protect me. Knowing this gives me great comfort and allows me to rest well and get a good night's sleep. Dear Lord, I affirm and remind myself that You are with me at all times and that I am safe in Your loving care. Grant me the serenity I need to rest easy, knowing that You are with me every step of the way, even when I slumber. I command the cares of the day to melt away as I lay down to sleep, and my spirit will find peace in Your presence. My spirit,

Unlock Deep Sleep Secrets

body, and mind need a good night's sleep, so I decree that My spirit, body, and mind will get a good night's sleep in Jesus' name. I will not be afraid of the night, because Lord Jesus, You are my refuge and strength. I declare it so in Jesus' name. Amen.

31 Days to Overcoming Insomnia

JOURNAL
"Sound Sleep is Important"

Morning Cognitive Renewal Statements

- Today, peace flows into me because I trust His unfailing protection.
- This morning, I will clothe myself in faith, not in fear.
- My mind is renewed, my heart is steady, and I begin today covered by grace

Morning Mindful Rest Practices

- **Mental Reset Practice:** Sit quietly for 1 minute. Inhale slowly and say in your mind: *"In peace."* Exhale slowly and say: *"...I dwell in safety."* Repeat for 3–5 breaths. Imagine yourself placing the worries or unfinished tasks of yesterday into God's hands. Whisper: *"Lord, I release what is behind me."*

- **Reset for Today:** Say aloud: "Because You protected me through the night, I walk in peace today." NOW, visualize yourself stepping into the day clothed in His grace and shielded by His protection.

Morning Journal Guided Reflections

Reflect on how God's protection gave you peace through the night. Write down one way you experienced His care while you rested, and one way you will trust His covering as you step into today?

_____
_____
_____
_____
_____

Evening Cognitive Renewal Statements

- Tonight, I am safe because the Lord surrounds me with His protection.
- His grace is my covering; His love is my shield.
- God's faithfulness ends my day in peace and begins my tomorrow in strength.

Evening Mindful Rest Practices

Before bed, sit quietly for 5 minutes. Reflect on your day, and with each deep breath, release one concern into God's care. Whisper Psalm 4:8: *"In peace I will lie down and sleep, for You*

Unlock Deep Sleep Secrets

alone, Lord, make me dwell in safety." As you exhale, picture God's faithfulness wrapping around you like a shield, ending your day in peace.

Evening Journal Guided Reflections

Write down three ways God's grace protected or sustained you today, big or small. End your list with the declaration: *"God's faithfulness ends my day in peace and begins my tomorrow in strength.*

Day 3
ADJUST YOUR MENTAL FREQUENCY

Philippians 4:8 (KJV):
"Finally, brethren, whatsoever things are true, whatsoever things are honest, whatsoever things are just, whatsoever things are pure, whatsoever things are lovely, whatsoever things are of good report; if there be any virtue, and if there be any praise, think on these things."

Imagine this: You've been up all day, your body is sore, but your mind won't shut down. You have a million and one things in your mind—events to plan for, regrets to make, an endless laundry list. You shut your eyes and snooze, but the noise of your head increases. We're all susceptible to these psycho-storms sometimes, the fact of the matter. But what if I told you, you could alter your mind's frequency, that you could put your brain on a channel that enables calm, rest, and lucid sleep?

And yes, you heard that right: you can tune your brain. And the best part? You have control over it.

Your mind can be dialed to the frequency of calm, rest, and peace, like you dial a radio dial. It is the Bible that has given us the recipe to shift our mental beats, and it begins with a strong verse: Philippians 4:8 (NIV): *"So lastly brothers and sisters, whatever is true, whatever is honorable, whatever is good, whatever is clean, whatever is beautiful, whatever is admirable, if anything is great or good, think of it."*

It's not just a tip—it's an injunction, and it tells you to bring your mind into the place where peace and clarity will be. Just imagine the possibilities: if you listen to these loving, upbeat frequencies, your mind will no longer chatter away and you will be able to get the restful sleep you are craving.

Unlock Deep Sleep Secrets

Let's jump right in and see how you can tune your mental frequency to get started with deep sleep.

The Power of Your Mental Frequency

Have you ever wondered if what your mind thinks is determining how you feel and how active you are? When you go to bed thinking about a stressful event, the rest of your day is brushstrokes in that same frantic ink. And it's the same thing if you lay down in bed with all the things that happened or will happen tomorrow, then you cannot go to sleep. Your mind frequency carries you into the world.

Consider this now if you adjust that frequency. If you intentionally choose to live by what is good, true, pure, beautiful and wonderful, you literally rewire your mind. You open up the door to tranquility. And harmony is the bedrock of slumber.

The Battle for Your Thoughts

Before we go into the glitz, the answer, let's first identify the battle in your head. You have two options each night, when getting ready for bed: you can stay or you can go.

The Distraction – The internal chaos of anxieties, complaints, and uncertainties. It is the river of tension and mess that keeps you up at night. The mind might be racing and spinning so much it isn't relaxing.

The Power of Peace – The peaceful channel that's in silence. It's a sound populated by ideas of thanksgiving, faith, and the beauty of God's Word. It's the station you have to be on to fall asleep.

But the trick is, YOU ARE THE DIAL OPERATOR.

You can switch the station. And you can choose, free of charge, to LISTEN to ideas about sleep and quiet.

How to Get Your Mind in The Swing: How to Do It Step-by-Step

But how do you adjust your mental frequency? Let's break it down into small bites you can do today to make your bedtime a little bit easier and let the serenity of deep sleep enter your home.

1. Recognize the Noise
Begin by taking responsibility for what's occurring in your head. Are you obsessed about something that happened during the day? Are you up at night worrying about tomorrow? The way to clean it is by identifying the mental mess. Awareness is the key.

31 Days to Overcoming Insomnia

2. Focus on What Is True – Turn Your Attention to What Is True
Philippians 4:8 opens with "whatever is true." Get real. Not scared. Where are you in life? Maybe you were down today but hey, you survived. Maybe you don't know what's next but hey, you're not alone. Tomorrow's a day you are equipped to confront.

3. Embrace the Pure and Lovely
So while your mind is already asleep, consider what is lovely and pure. What brings you joy? An image, a scene, a verse to reaffirm? Go there in your mind. Imagine being somewhere in nature, perhaps by a calm lake or in a garden that's in full bloom. Fill your mind with beauty.

4. Practice Gratitude
Gratitude helps to tune you out in your mind. Before you go to bed, ask God to bless your day with many blessings, big and small. And thank Him for the rest He's going to give you, and for the energy you had today, and for the calm He gives you amid the storm. Gratitude is a game-changer.

5. Release Control
There is always mental mess from the balancing act. And here's the thing, you don't need to be an expert yet. Don't worry and let God handle it. You don't have to be a slave to tomorrow's woes today. Don't do it. Allow yourself to believe it's all going to be fine. Let God carry the burden. Rest in His promises.

6. Meditate on God's Peace
And lastly, finish the day by spending time in God's Word. Philippians 4:8 gives us a whopping list of attributes to aim for, but here's another one to add to your list: *"You will keep in perfect peace those whose hearts are unshaken because they put their hope in you."* (Isaiah 26:3). Put God's calm on your back as you drift off to sleep. Just remember He is watching over you and you will be at His complete peace.

The Ripple Effect of Changing Your Mental Frequency
And here's the kicker: When you change your frequency, not only will you start sleeping better your whole life changes, too. The rest you feel extends into your friends, your career, and your life outlook. The more you decide to stay in the beautiful, the authentic, and the excellent, the more calm will prevail over your days and nights.

And as your brain frequency changes, you'll start to sleep without thinking. You'll fall asleep much more readily into the type of restful sleep your body and mind desperately need to recharge. And you will come out of bed energized, restored, and equipped to face the day with renewed calm and clarity.

Unlock Deep Sleep Secrets

The Power Is in Your Hands
This is the good news: you are not helpless in this fight for sleep. You can switch the frequency of your mind any time. And God's will is for you to think things that will bring you rest, joy, and sleep.

And when you heed Philippians 4:8, the more you tune your mind in the direction of all that is true, lovely, pure, and praiseworthy, the more rest you will experience—that deep, rejuvenating sleep that you've been craving.

Peace isn't something that you get but rather something you decide. So next time you lay your head down tonight, relax. Choose rest. Adjust your mind speed and sleep like you were born to do so.

YOU HOLD THE DIAL. TUNE IN TO PEACE. SLEEP WELL!

Prayer for the Journey
Dear God, You are a loving Father, I come to You tonight with my mind and heart filled with many thoughts. I thank You for the instruction You have given me in Philippians 4:8 to focus on whatever is true, noble, just, pure, lovely, and praiseworthy. I confess that, too often, my thoughts stray towards worry, fear, or negativity, which keeps me from experiencing Your peace and restful sleep.

Lord, help me to meditate on Your truth as I prepare to rest. Guide my thoughts to dwell on Your goodness, Your faithfulness, and Your love. Let my mind be filled with things that are noble and pure, things that reflect Your character. As I think on these things, calm my spirit and let Your peace guard my heart and mind. I release every worry and every fear into Your hands, trusting that You are in control. Thank You, Lord, for the gift of peaceful sleep.

Tonight, I choose to rest in the truth that You are my provider, my protector, and my peace. Let me fall asleep with my thoughts centered on You, and may I wake up refreshed, renewed, and ready to face the new day. I trust in Your care, knowing that Your peace surpasses all understanding and will guide me through the night. In Jesus' name. Amen.

31 Days to Overcoming Insomnia

JOURNAL

"Sound Sleep is Important"

Morning Cognitive Renewal Statements

- Today, I choose to focus on what is good and true. I will think on things that bring me peace, joy, and encouragement. I will not let negative thoughts take control of my mind.
- I control my mental channel. I align my thoughts with God's truth, and I fill my mind with what is pure, lovely, and praiseworthy.

Morning Mindful Rest Practices

- **Mental Reset Practice:** When you wake up, spend 5 minutes in quiet reflection. Identify any lingering negative or anxious thoughts, then intentionally "change the channel" by thinking of something good, true, or lovely. Repeat Philippians 4:8 aloud and visualize yourself switching to a peaceful mental state.
- **Positive Thought Journaling:** Start your day by writing down three positive, uplifting thoughts or things you are grateful for. This practice helps set the tone for your day and encourages a mindset of positivity and peace.

    - _____
    - _____
    - _____

Morning Journal Guided Reflections

What thoughts occupy my mind as I start the day?
_____
_____
_____
_____

Are they in line with Philippians 4:8?
_____
_____
_____
_____

Unlock Deep Sleep Secrets

How can I intentionally focus on positive, life-giving thoughts today?
_____
_____
_____

Evening Cognitive Renewal Statements

- As I prepare for sleep, I release all thoughts that do not serve me. I choose to think on what is true, noble, and lovely. My mind is at peace, and I rest in God's truth.
- I shift my thoughts to what brings me joy and peace. I let go of negativity and embrace God's goodness. I sleep peacefully, knowing that my mind is focused on Him.

Evening Mindful Rest Practices

Mental Detox: Before bed, reflect on the thoughts that have occupied your mind throughout the day. Are they in line with Philippians 4:8?
_____
_____
_____

If your thoughts were not in line with the verse, take a moment to identify and "switch" those thoughts by focusing on something praiseworthy. Speak aloud the positive thoughts you want to dwell on before sleep.

Evening Journal Guided Reflections

What mental "channels" do I need to change before I go to sleep?
_____
_____
_____

What praiseworthy or lovely thoughts can I meditate on tonight to bring peace and rest?
_____
_____
_____

31 Days to Overcoming Insomnia

Gratitude Reflection

It is important that you focus on positive aspects of your day, so you can shift your mind away from worry and into a state of peace, which is essential for restful sleep.

Write down three things from the day that were lovely.

- I am grateful for_____
- I am thankful for _____
- I appreciate for _____

Write down three things from the day that were admirable.

- I am grateful for_____
- I am thankful for _____
- I appreciate for _____

Write down three things from the day that were praiseworthy.

- I am grateful for_____
- I am thankful for _____
- I appreciate for _____

Mindful Rest Practices

Continue with what you have learned on this day for one week. Then respond to the following questions about what you have experienced.

How has changing my mental channel affected my sleep and my overall mindset?
_____
_____
_____

Where have I noticed the most improvement in my thought life?
_____
_____
_____

Day 4
DIGITAL DETOX: RECLAIMING PEACE FROM SCREENS

Psalm 101:3 (ESV):
*"I will not set before my eyes anything that is worthless.
I hate the work of those who fall away; it shall not cling to me."*

Suppose: You have been up all day, your mind has taken up the place of sleep, and you're ready to close your eyes, to get into the twilight sleep your body needs. But then, the temptation hits. You check your phone, social media, emails. You look back, and an hour later your eyes are dry, and your brain is in overdrive. Sound familiar?

If we live a life in front of screens, it is all too easy to become immersed in digital overload. From social media to business emails, from scrolling through mindless images, information overload steals our time and keeps us up at night. But here's the thing: You can take your peace back. And it starts with an online cleanse.

We're going to look at how avoiding screens, especially before bedtime, can make a big difference in how your mind is clearer, your mind feels calmer, and your sleep becomes deeper and more restful. You'll be taught to unplug, reboot, and get back that peace and silence your soul is longing for.

Let's dive in.

The Internet Puzzle: Screens Take Our Hearts in Their Hands

It is a "plugged-in" world. All the pings, push notifications, and digital device notifications can become overwhelming. We are hooked to a perpetual cycle of data, opinion, and noise. Technological innovation isn't all good, and it's not all bad, either: it steals our solitude, robs our sleep, and makes our brains constantly on high alert.

31 Days to Overcoming Insomnia

Here's the Problem
We never had brains able to cope with all the information that is currently flowing into them. Researchers have documented that blue light from screens interrupts sleep, while the mind chatter of browsing social media or email continues even when we shut down the screen.

There's a reason why we sleep badly, too. We're overstimulated constantly and when we need to take a break, we can't turn it off.

Digital Detox Call: Our Time to Decode
The answer is clear, but deep: Get away from the monitors. A digital detox is just that, a deliberate, sanitized exhale from technicolor noise. We detox ourselves from screens—especially at night, to get our serenity back, our mind straight and we can get a good night's sleep.

Psalm 101:3 serves as an inspiration in this digital age: *"I will set nothing wicked before my eyes; I hate the work of those who fall away; it shall not cling to me."*

And this is the great teaching in this verse, that we have choices of what we put in our heads and heart. If we are choosy about the people and forces that we welcome into our homes, we should also be choosy about what we see on screen. If it is making us anxious, comparison, and/or disturbed, we can switch it off and keep our sanity. A digital detox means being in charge of what you're letting in, giving your brain some space, and settling for silence instead of bustle.

The Impact of Screens on Your Sleep
We can learn more about digital detox below but first, a quick explanation of the screen impact on your sleep. The ripples are massive, and the cure is in your grasp:

Blue Light Disrupts Melatonin Production
Blue light, from cellphones, tablets and computers, knocks out melatonin, the sleep hormone. When we're in the blue light – and, by extension, especially at night – our brains are lost, and it takes a long time for us to fall asleep.

Mental Stimulation Keeps You Alert
After you put down your phone, your brain doesn't sleep. The brain demands focus while you're scrolling through social media or reading a raging news headline, and it's difficult for your mind to quieten. You don't relax, but your brain is ablaze with new ideas, fears, and facts.

Unlock Deep Sleep Secrets

Disconnection from Reality
Screens also skew our reality. This perpetual comparing with others, these planned lives on the internet, this tsunami of data can be stressful, anxiety-producing, and self-doubting. There is a lot of cognitive noise which can be very hard to settle into.

How to Reclaim Your Peace: Steps for a Digital Detox
Now, let's get practical. Get your head back and your sleep back. How you can start a digital detox:

Set Boundaries for Screen Time
The first thing to do is define a timeframe for when you're done with screens. One of the best things you can do is to shut down all your screens at least 30 minutes before bed. This leaves your brain time to relax, wind down and get ready for bed. You can scroll but instead, read a book, write in a journal or listen to soothing music.

Create a Screen-Free Zone
Make your bedroom a sleeping space. Don't leave your phone, tablet, or computer in the room (or at least out of bed). If you wake up using your phone as an alarm, get an actual alarm clock. If you can keep screens out of the room, temptation will be dispelled, and you'll be able to have an overall quiet space to rest.

Curate Your Content
Not all screen time is bad. Social media and news are overwhelming, but there are lots of things you can consume that are good and positive. Subscribe to accounts that push you, uplift you, encourage you. Make sure you select something that will take your mind off of it. We can 'not look with approval' on that which disturbs our quiet, quoting Psalm 101:3. If you are feeling anxious or stressed by scrolling through certain apps, unfollow, unmute or redefine boundaries.

Restore Mindfulness in the Place of Screen Time
As a change, don't reach for your phone, pick something to do in the name of quiet and relaxation. Attempt some light stretching, herbal tea, prayer, or meditation. Or you can also take time to write in a gratitude journal about your day or read a Bible chapter. The more time you dispense with screen time in favor of mindful, calming activities, the more effortless it becomes to unwind.

Establish a Digital Sabbath
The best way to reboot your relationship with technology is by taking a 'digital Sabbath". A single day in a week, when you completely unplugged from all the screens. This is a time to get back in the dirt, with nature, your family, and with yourself. This digital cleanse can give you habits that will last for mental and sleep health.

31 Days to Overcoming Insomnia

The Advantages of a Digital Detox
Breaking from screens is good for you both now and later.

- ***Better Sleep:*** If you don't scroll before bed, your brain will relax and go to sleep much quicker and deeper.
- ***Less Stress & Anxiety:*** By detoxing from the digital junk, you eliminate the mental chatter that contributes to stress and anxiety.
- ***Better Focus and Clarity:*** When you have less screen time, you will regain mental clarity and get to the heart of your life.
- ***Rest in God and In Yourself:*** The quiet, no screens are time to rest in God and remember His peace. Unplugging will reveal that You Can Hear You More Well.

Making Peace, One Day at a Time
There is too much that matters to your well-being to be lost in screens. Time to stand up, put down your gun, and find your calm with a digital detox. It all starts with intentional choices—with what you let in your head, what you focus on, and what you disconnect from.

For when you do these things, always keep Psalm 101:3 in mind, that you guard your heart and your mind and that you never let anything that is evil and troublesome reside in your life. You can be still, or not; you can get out of your stuff and back in your stuff.

So, go ahead. Take a break from the screens. You will be rewarded in mind, body, and spirit. Your sleep will thank you. And you'll find the serenity you've been missing, one digital cleanse at a time.

Prayer for the Journey
Dear God, I praise you for Your mercy and the calm that comes to those who align their lives with Your will. Before I lay down tonight, I ask for Your empowerment to pursue a heart that is righteous. I unplug the chains of screen and digital devices that have seized my thoughts and focus for the day. Give me the strength and counsel to set no wicked thing before my eyes. I decree that no harmful influences will upset my spirit and draw me away from You. Teach me to filter out toxic influences so I can create an atmosphere of peace, making it easier to experience restful sleep and mental clarity.

I declare my heart and mind is purified from all that brings conflict. I make you Lord in my house so let Your presence permeate this environment, my home which is my place of rest and security. As I lay to sleep, I declare my thoughts are pure, lovely and worthy of praise. Lord, please keep my mind and heart as I pull down strongholds and bring every thought to the obedience of Jesus Christ. In Jesus' name. Amen.

Unlock Deep Sleep Secrets

JOURNAL
"Sound Sleep is Important"

Our minds need time to unplug from the distractions of the day. Reducing screen time before bed is a powerful way to prepare for restful sleep. By practicing a nightly digital detox, we honor our bodies' need for rest and our spirits' need for stillness. In this space of calm, we can more easily hear God's voice and feel His peace. The activity below will aid you in detoxing.

Mindful Rest Practices: Digital Detox Before Bed

- **Setting the Intention**
- **Time**: 15-30 minutes before bed
- **What You'll Need**: A quiet space, your Bible, and a journal

Step 1: Reflect on Psalm 101:3

Begin by reading Psalm 101:3: *"I will not set before my eyes anything that is worthless."* Reflect on the meaning of this verse in today's context. Consider the content you consume through your phone, TV, or computer—are these things that promote peace and spiritual well-being, or do they leave you feeling anxious, distracted, or empty?

_____
_____
_____
_____
_____
_____
_____

Journal Prompt: What are the "worthless" things you may be setting before your eyes? How does the content you consume before bed affect your mind and heart? Write down your thoughts.

_____
_____
_____
_____
_____
_____
_____

31 Days to Overcoming Insomnia

Step 2: Disconnect from Devices
For the next 15-30 minutes before bed, commit to a digital detox. Turn off your phone, tablet, and computer, and place them in a different room or set them to "Do Not Disturb" mode. Resist the urge to check messages or scroll through social media.

Step 3: Engage in a Screen-Free Activity
Instead of reaching for your phone, use this time to calm your mind and prepare for rest. Choose one or more of the following screen-free activities:

- **Read Scripture or Devotional**: Pick a calming scripture, such as Psalm 23 or Psalm 91, and meditate on it. Let the words bring peace to your spirit and invite God's presence into your evening.
- **Journal**: Write down any lingering thoughts, worries, or reflections from your day. This helps clear your mind before bed, ensuring that these thoughts don't keep you awake later.
- **Practice Gratitude**: In your journal, write down three things you are grateful for from the day. This practice shifts your focus away from distractions and stress, grounding you in positivity and peace.
- **Reflect on God's Creation**: Take a few moments to sit in silence or step outside briefly if possible. Focus on the sounds of nature or the calmness of the night. Let this moment of quiet be a reminder of God's presence and the beauty of His creation.

Journal Prompt: After unplugging from your devices and engaging in a calming activity, how do you feel compared to nights when you used electronics right up until bed? Did you notice a difference in your mental state or mood?

_____
_____
_____
_____
_____
_____
_____
_____
_____
_____
_____
_____
_____
_____
_____
_____
_____
_____

Unlock Deep Sleep Secrets

Step 4: Prayer for Peaceful Rest
Close your evening by offering a prayer for rest, asking God to guard your heart and mind as you sleep. You can use this simple prayer or create one of your own:

"Lord, I surrender this day into Your hands. I lay aside every distraction and worry, and I ask for Your peace to cover me as I sleep. Help me to keep my eyes on what is true, lovely, and worthy, and guide my heart away from what is unworthy. Thank You for Your presence, Your protection, and Your peace. Amen."

Journal Prompt: After several nights of digital detox, reflect on how it has affected your sleep quality and overall sense of peace. What habits or distractions could you adjust in your daily life to help you keep your focus on things that are spiritually enriching?

_____
_____
_____
_____
_____
_____
_____
_____
_____
_____
_____

Practical Tips for Digital Detox Success:

- **Establish a Screen-Free Zone**: Keep electronic devices out of your bedroom to create a restful environment that's free from digital distractions.
- **Set a "No Screen" Rule Before Bed**: Commit to unplugging from all screens at least 30 minutes before bed. Use this time to read, reflect, pray, or engage in a relaxing, non-digital activity.
- **Use Analog Tools**: Switch to using an old-fashioned alarm clock instead of your phone and keep a physical Bible or devotional book by your bed for evening reflection.
- **Track Your Progress**: Use your journal to track how your digital detox has affected your sleep and mental well-being over time. Celebrate small victories as you form healthier habits.

Day 5
SLEEP AND MENTAL HEALTH: REST FOR THE MIND AND SPIRIT

Matthew 11:28-30 (NKJV):
"Come to Me, all you who labor and are heavy laden, and I will give you rest. Take My yoke upon you and learn from Me, for I am gentle and lowly in heart, and you will find rest for your souls. For My yoke is easy and My burden is light."

And we all know how it feels, those nights when you can't get any sleep at all. You are groggy, your body is crying sleep, but your mind is not. Ideas are going around and around. Tomorrow's fears, yesterday's regrets, list after list and everything in between blow like a hurricane in your head. You are in a downslide by the load of all of it, unable to get the rest your body and soul desperately desire.

But what if I showed you that sleep is deeply related to mental health—and that, with the care of your mind and spirit, you can find the restorative sleep you have been missing?

Sleep isn't just an actual physical necessity, but a mental and spiritual one. Rest your brain and soul as much as your body. And the wonderful part is, God allows us to have that rest.

Let's dig in and find out how sleep can help heal your mind, body and soul —and how with God's Word, you can start feeling the peace that comes from rest.

The Relationship Between Sleep and Mood Disorder
We may imagine sleep as simply physical: our bodies' recharge—but that's also true for mental health. Actually, sleep deprivation or bad sleep ruins your mind and your heart, making you irritable, anxious, depressed, and unable to concentrate or think properly.

Unlock Deep Sleep Secrets

And here's why sleep and mental health are so close:

Sleep Recharges Your Brain
Your brain cleans itself and recharges during deep sleep—all the waste products from daytime brain firing is removed, leaving your mind sharp and clear. You just can't do this properly without enough rest, and your brain gets all confused and stressed. That causes mental exhaustion, crankiness, and even mood swings.

Sleep Helps Regulate Emotions
It takes sleep to regulate the emotions. When we are not sleeping enough, our emotional centers begin to overreact. Little irritations turn into massive ones, and the resilience to stress suffers. In contrast, a good night's sleep makes us better at taking on difficulties with more grace and grit, so we can enter the day with a more focused and calmer mind.

Sleep Aids in Developing Mental Clarity and Decision-Making
An alert brain makes better decisions, problem-solves better, and thinks better. We have reduced rational judgment, and the most basic things can become overwhelming if we're sleep-deprived. This is all stress and anxiety, wherein being not able to sleep adds to the difficulties.

The Activation of Sleep in the Soul
Sleep is not only physical and mental, but spiritual as well. God made us to sleep. Indeed, God Himself was the model of rest in the Bible when He made the world. Six days of work and He slept the seventh. But why? Was He tired? No—He slept so that we can learn the value of rest in every field. God is a good sleeper. And just like your body and brain need to sleep, so should your soul.

The Call to Rest: Matthew 11:28-30
Jesus in the Gospel of Matthew 11:28-30 (NIV) offers a lovely invitation to everyone who is tired and burdened: *"Come to me, all you who labor and are heavy-laden, and I will make ye sleep. So, learn from me, yea, be taught of me, since I am mild-hearted and lowly in heart, and your souls shall be at ease. My burden is light and my burden easy."*

These passages are God's invocation for rest—not just body rest, but soul rest. It's easy to get bogged down in a maelstrom of demands and stresses in this world. But Jesus says let us lay them down and rest in Him.

When we relinquish our fears and worries to God, God does more than just give us a night's rest physically—He gives us a night's rest for our souls. Such sleep is a breath of silence for the mind, a cure for the soul, and a rest for the body.

31 Days to Overcoming Insomnia

The Strength of Rest for Your Mind: The Miracle of Rest
When your mind and heart are placed in the Lord, the payoff is great. Deep sleep brings mental focus, emotional stability, and spiritual tranquility. With the beginning of soul resting, you will see the stress and anxiety melt away; your mind becomes clearer and more relaxed.

You can go through the day more with a bit more energy, grace, and happiness. There is no longer a physiological need for sleep; now there is a spiritual one—to leave your troubles at the door and open yourself up to the peace of God.

Resting in God's Peace
Not only do you sleep to rest your body, but you sleep for your mind and soul as well. When you allow rest for your soul, you invite renewal. And God's invitation to sleep tells us we needn't go through it alone. If we have faith in Him and put aside our anxieties, then restorative sleep is the peace and stillness we need.

So when you're going to bed tonight, keep these lovely words in mind—Matthew 11:28-30. Come to Jesus—give away all that you have and let Him take care of your soul. Rest in His peace. He will renew your mind and spirit with His healing hand and tomorrow, you will be able to get up again reformed and refreshed ready to take Him for all He has for you.

Sleep is not sleep, but an invitation to lie in the arms of the One who brings peace which is unmatchable. And that is sleep for the soul.

Prayer for the Journey
Dear God, I come before You, resting in Your promise according to Matthew 11:28-30. I am giving all my worries, anxiety, fears, and burdens to You. I carry worry, anxiety, and fears because of physical exhaustion, emotional strain, and spiritual heaviness. I surrender my mind and heart to You tonight.

Jesus, You said **"Come unto me,"** *so I am coming to You in simple trust and surrender. I want to have a wonderful relationship and build intimacy with You.*

Jesus, You said, **"Take my yoke upon you"** *just like a yoke is placed on an ox to share the load. Thank you for promising to walk alongside me to help carry my burdens daily. I want to learn from You and follow Your ways. Your* **yoke is easy and Your burden is light** *because Your teachings bring peace and freedom.*

Let Your presence cover me like a hen covers her chicks, guiding my sleep.

Tonight, I receive Your promise of rest. Thank you for Your unwavering love and for providing the peaceful rest I need tonight. In Jesus name. Amen.

Unlock Deep Sleep Secrets

JOURNAL
"Sound Sleep is Important"

Mindful Rest Practices: Releasing Your Mental Burdens to Christ

Breathing in Peace, Breathing Out Burdens
One way to calm the mind and prepare it for rest is through deep, focused breathing. This exercise helps you center your thoughts on Christ and His promise of rest, while letting go of the burdens that weigh you down.

Step 1: Find a Comfortable Position
Sit or lie down in a comfortable position, making sure you're in a quiet space where you won't be disturbed.

Step 2: Begin with Deep Breaths
Slowly inhale through your nose, filling your lungs completely, and then exhale slowly through your mouth. With each inhale, focus on the words of Jesus: *"Come to me, all you who are weary..."* Imagine the peace of Christ filling you with each breath. As you exhale, imagine releasing your burdens and worries into His hands. Continue this for several minutes.

Step 3: Meditate on Matthew 11:28-30
As you continue your breathing, meditate on Matthew 11:28-30. Let the image of Jesus offering you rest sink into your heart. Picture yourself exchanging your heavy burdens for His light yoke, one filled with grace, peace, and gentleness.

Journal Guided Reflections

After your breathing exercise, how did you feel?

_____
_____
_____

Did focusing on Jesus' invitation to rest help calm your mind? What burdens did you feel yourself releasing?

_____
_____
_____

31 Days to Overcoming Insomnia

Prayer for Mental Rest

Often, the burdens that affect our mental health are too heavy to carry alone. This prayer exercise focuses on releasing your mental burdens to Christ, trusting Him to carry what you cannot.

Step 1: Identify Your Burdens

Before bed, take a moment to reflect on the thoughts, worries, or stresses that are weighing heavily on your mind. Write them down in your journal. Be specific—whether it's work-related stress, relationship issues, health concerns, or general anxiety, acknowledge these burdens.

Step 2: Pray Over Each Burden

For each burden, offer a simple prayer of surrender, like:
"Lord, I give You this burden of (name your specific worry). I lay it at Your feet, trusting in Your promise to give me rest. Help me to release this burden into Your hands, knowing that Your yoke is easy, and Your burden is light."

Step 3: Rest in His Promise

As you finish your prayer, take a moment of stillness, breathing in the peace that Jesus offers. Trust that He is carrying your burdens and let go of the need to hold onto them.

Journal Guided Reflections

How did you feel after praying over your burdens?

_____
_____
_____
_____

Were you able to surrender your worries to Jesus? Did this help prepare your mind for rest?

_____
_____
_____
_____

Progressive Muscle Relaxation to Ease Mental Tension

Mental health challenges can cause physical tension in the body, and this tension can make it hard to relax and fall asleep. Progressive muscle relaxation is a simple exercise that helps ease both physical and mental stress by focusing on one muscle group at a time.

Unlock Deep Sleep Secrets

Step 1: Focus on Your Body
Begin by lying down comfortably in your bed. Close your eyes and take a few deep breaths to center yourself.

Step 2: Tense and Release
Starting with your feet, tense the muscles in your toes for 5-10 seconds, and then release. Move to your legs, then your stomach, arms, shoulders, and finally, your neck. With each release, imagine letting go of the mental tension and stress you've been carrying.

Step 3: Combine with Scripture
As you work through each muscle group, quietly repeat the words of Matthew 11:30: "For my yoke is easy, and my burden is light." With each release, visualize Christ lifting your burdens, giving you both physical and mental rest.

Journal Prompt: After practicing progressive muscle relaxation, how did your body feel? Did the physical release of tension help quiet your mind? How did focusing on the words of Matthew 11:30 affect your sense of peace?

Guided Reflection

Mental health challenges like stress, anxiety, and depression can rob us of rest, both physically and spiritually. But Jesus' promise in Matthew 11:28-30 is an invitation to come to Him when we are weary and weighed down. By focusing on His promise of rest, we can let go of the burdens that trouble our minds, allowing ourselves to rest in His presence.

Incorporating practices like deep breathing, prayer, and physical relaxation into your nightly routine can help ease mental and emotional tension, creating space for the deep rest that Christ offers. When we release our mental burdens to Him, we not only improve our sleep, but also experience the soul-level peace He promises.

Journal Guided Reflections
Reflect on how your mental health has affected your sleep. What specific burdens or worries keep you awake at night?

_____
_____
_____
_____

How does turning to Christ in prayer, breathing exercises, and relaxation help calm your mind?

_____
_____
_____
_____

31 Days to Overcoming Insomnia

How to Get Ahead with Your Sleep and Mental Health:

- Establish a Relaxing Nighttime Schedule: Before going to bed, prayer, meditation, and reflection are time for moving from day-to-day stress into relaxation.
- Avoid Stimulants: Avoid caffeine, alcohol, and late-night meals as these can make you anxious or interfere with your sleep.
- Move: Physical activities throughout the day can make you more sleep-ready as well as mentally fit by easing stress levels and improving mood.
- Find Community Support: If the psychiatric issues are getting to you, consult with a counselor, close friend, or spiritual authority.

Day 6
INSOMNIA IS FROM HELL:
BREAKING FREE FROM SLEEPLESSNESS

Leviticus 26:6 (NIV):
"I will grant peace in the land, and you will lie down,
and no one will make you afraid. I will remove wild beasts from the land,
and the sword will not pass through your country."

Consider the following scenario: You have just been through an exhausting day. Your body is sore, you're exhausted, and you aren't sleeping when you lift your head off the pillow. You toss and turn. You go a few hours, and your brain just goes racing. Nervousness, anxiety, stress, and fear just come down like flood water keeping you up at night when you just want to sleep. Sound familiar?

Not only is it an annoyance, but it's also a spiritual struggle. Not only is insomnia a form of sleeplessness, but it can also be a weapon the enemy has to take your peace, your happiness, and your health. The never-ending rhythm of inertia can exhaust you mentally, emotionally and spiritually. But here is the secret for you: God doesn't give you insomnia. Actually, it begins with the enemy trying to prevent you from living out the abundant life God has for you, and that includes some wholesome, rejuvenating sleep.

Let's learn about the manifestation of insomnia as a spiritual derangement, understand the root of insomnia, and break free from sleeplessness with the promise of rest and peace that God has given us. You don't belong to the sleepless night. When God's Word is your hammer, you can get back your rest and your tranquility.

Understanding the Enemy's Tactics
Sleep can sometimes be a dark side, one that sneaks in, out of the blue, disrupting your mind, body, and soul. If sleep is a no-go, it's like you're on the losing side. But the Bible says

31 Days to Overcoming Insomnia

God does not make confusion or disorder—it is the enemy who makes that happen.

Consider Leviticus 26:6 (NIV): Look at these words:
"I will make the earth tranquil, and ye shall lie down and nobody shall scare you. I will take away wild animals from the land, and the sword will not come in your land."

This is a very powerful word; it's a word of God's rest. When we are right with Him, He rests us, not merely for the flesh, but also for the soul. Nightmares, and their worrying and aversive night's sleep, aren't God's. It's the symptom of something else, an uphill battle for your solitude and your mind. The devil knows that if he can keep you awake, then he can leave you vulnerable. He lives for disturbance. and insomnia is one of his favorite tricks to strip you of the rest and happiness God wants for you.

The Spiritual Roots of Insomnia

Most of the time, insomnia is not an irritable brain or caffeine high—it's a demonic attack. If we're tired, frail, or just feeling overwhelmed, the enemy wants to take advantage of that frailty, so he arouses fear and anxiety in our brains. These psychiatric battles stir the night with our bodies unsettling and confused.

Night terrors, aversion, and unforgiveness can make insomnia possible—as if fear or unresolved feelings are mental walls of which we sleep. In fear of the future, guilt about the past, and anxiety about the present, if our mind is wracked with a storm, we cannot sleep. These fortresses are exploited by the enemy, and this is even harder to reconcile.

It is in such times that we need to remember that God has not given us a spirit of fear, but of power, love and of the good will (2 Timothy 1:7). Fear, anxiety, and insomnia: these are the devil's tools in our servitude. But God's Word says we will be free, and we will be at peace, and we will be at rest.

The Power of God's Peace

When we put God into the bed with us, it is because God is master. God is a peacemaker and wants His children to have peace every part of our lives—sleep being no exception. In placing our anxieties in His hands, we lay them open to His love which is greater than all knowledge. This quiet is an act of God that calms our heart and minds, even in calamity.

Our need for rest is brought directly from Leviticus 26:6 – and what a promise it is:
I will give you rest on the land, and you will lie down and nobody shall terrorize you.
This is not just a physical peace; it's a mind-protecting peace. You will be able to sleep in the night because God's quiet is guarding you. You will have no rogue animal (dread or fear) disturbing your sleep, and no sword (the attacks of the adversary) injuring your heart.

Unlock Deep Sleep Secrets

Free from Sleepless Nights: How-To Tips to Get to Sleep Peacefully
But how do we resist insomnia and reclaim the night of sleep God had left for us? These are some actionable things you can do to stop waking up late:

Pray for Peace
Pray when the nighttime terror sets in and you start to feel nervous. Don't fight the good fight on your own; go to God, the greatest savior. Call upon Him and have Him put you to rest and only His peace can give. *"In peace I will lie down and sleep, for you alone, Lord, make me dwell in safety,"* Psalm 4:8 tells us. Ask God to bring you that peace as you invite Him into your trials.

Release Your Worries
Sleep is like soil of concern. When you go to bed at night, surrender your anxieties to God. Copy them out if you must and hand them over in prayer. Tell yourself that God is in charge and that everything else is in His hands. When you stop trying to be in charge, your mind will settle.

God's Word: Speak Over Your Sleep
God's Word has its veto over insomnia. Declare the scripture aloud before bed. Say, "I will lay down and sleep in safety, because only You, Lord, keep me therein safe" (Psalm 4:8). Speak to the dread, the anxiety, and the anxious with the voice of God's Word. God is faithful. He will set you on a stable foundation.

Create a Restful Environment
Mood: Sleeping depends on the atmosphere. Create a space in your bedroom that is a haven for tranquility. Refrain from turning screens on, turn the lights down, and just keep your environment quiet as possible. Try aromatherapy like lavender or soothing music to keep things calm. The more peaceful your environment, the more quickly you fall asleep.

Trust in God's Sovereignty
Just trust God is in charge. We are prone to insomnia if we are exhausted or run over. Feed God your worries and trust His sovereignty. He can give you a break to rest your weary soul. And if you can trust in His love and power than worry, then you can have rest.

The Victory Over Insomnia
Don't forget: Sleep isn't yours. It doesn't have to be you. All God wants for you is rest, peace, and an easy mind. Sleep is the enemy, out to seize your night and make you sleepy and agitated. But you can rouse from the bed of sleeplessness by the Word of God and His peace.

Jesus wrote in Matthew 11:28-30: *"Come to me, all you who are weary and heavy laden, and I will give you rest."* He said the same thing about every part of your life, including

31 Days to Overcoming Insomnia

sleep. He wants you to put your life on His lap, including your insomnia, and rely on Him for sleep.

When you let go and trust in His peace, and then do the work of healing, you will start sleeping well, for it is your inheritance as a child of God. Nightmares don't have to be your life. Be sure of God's Word and savor the repose that He has for you.

The fight for sleep is real, but the victory is not. Jesus gives you rest for your soul and that rest is restful sleep. No more sleepless nights, and no more worrying, because God is in your heart and mind.

Prayer for the Journey

Dear God, I come before you tonight declaring that You are the God of tranquility. <u>You promise to bless Your people with peace, security, and prosperity if they walk in Your ways.</u>

Your Word declares in Leviticus 26:6 says, "You will grant peace in the land, and that when I will lie down, and no one will make me afraid. You will remove wild beasts from the land, and the sword will not pass through my country."

Lord, You said, "I will give peace in the land and we shall lie down and none shall be afraid." Thank you for the promise of peace in my house tonight. A peace which comes from a deep sense of security and well-being. Lord, You said, "We will lie down and not be afraid." Therefore, I decree that I am in a state of restful trust and every external threat from negative invading thoughts are neutralized in Jesus' name. I curse fear, anxiety, and disturbances that seek to rob me of peaceful sleep. I trust You to guard my home, my mind, and my spirit from all harm just as You promise to rid the land of harmful beast and threats.

I remind myself that Your peace is not fragile but powerful – a peace that passed all understanding and it is able to guard my heart and mind.

Lord, I stand on Your promise and declare that insomnia, sleeplessness, and restlessness is not of You: therefore, it is broken in my life today in Jesus' name. I declare that sleep is my portion, and I cast out every fear and worry that seems to steal God's promise of sound sleep for Your beloved child.

According to Leviticus 26: 6, I decree that no wild beast of stress, panic, or any form of sleeplessness will come near my dwelling. I declare that I have sound sleep, and that God has already given me peace and I accept his promise. **In Jesus' name. Amen.**

Unlock Deep Sleep Secrets

JOURNAL
"Sound Sleep is Important"

Mindful Meditation to Ease Insomnia

Practicing mindfulness can help shift your focus away from the frustrations of insomnia and bring you into a peaceful, restful state. By meditating on God's promises, you can quiet your mind and body, inviting the Holy Spirit to calm your spirit.

Guided Reflections: Resting in God's Peace

1. **Prepare Your Space:** Find a comfortable, quiet place where you can relax. If you're in bed, make sure your surroundings are conducive to sleep (low lighting, minimal noise).
2. **Begin with Deep Breathing:** Inhale slowly for 4 counts, hold for 4 counts, and exhale for 6 counts. Repeat this breathing pattern several times, allowing your body to relax with each exhale.
3. **Focus on Leviticus 26:6:** As you continue to breathe deeply, repeat the words of the scripture to yourself: *"I will grant peace in the land, and you will lie down, and no one will make you afraid."* Imagine God speaking these words over you, granting peace in your body and mind. Picture yourself lying down in safety, free from fear or restlessness.
4. **Release Your Worries:** With each breath, mentally release any stress, anxiety, or burdens that are keeping you awake. As you exhale, imagine these worries floating away, replaced by God's peace. With each breath, feel your body becoming more relaxed and ready for rest.
5. **Visualize God's Protection:** Picture God's protective hand over you, keeping away the "wild beasts" of fear and sleeplessness. Feel His presence calming you and letting you drift into peaceful sleep

Guided Reflections to Explore Insomnia and Rest

Writing about your experience with insomnia can help you process the emotions and frustrations it brings. By journaling, you can reflect on what keeps you awake and how God's Word can restore your peace. Use these prompts to guide your reflections:

- What thoughts or concerns keep me awake at night?
  _____
  _____
  _____

31 Days to Overcoming Insomnia

- How does my struggle with sleep affect my emotional, physical, and spiritual well-being?

  _____
  _____
  _____
  _____

- In what ways does Leviticus 26:6 remind me that God desires peace and rest for me?

  _____
  _____
  _____
  _____

- How can I trust God to "remove the wild beasts" that disrupt my peace and sleep?

  _____
  _____
  _____
  _____

- What changes can I make in my evening routine to prepare my mind and heart for restful sleep?

  _____
  _____
  _____
  _____

Optional: As you breathe, meditate on Leviticus 26:6. Silently repeat the phrase, *"I will grant peace in the land, and you will lie down, and no one will make you afraid,"* allowing the truth of God's promise to sink into your mind and spirit.

Progressive Muscle Relaxation

This is another exercise that helps you release physical tension from your body, which often contributes to sleeplessness. Here's how to practice it:

- **Start with Your Feet**: Begin by tensing the muscles in your feet. Hold the tension for a few seconds, then release.

Unlock Deep Sleep Secrets

- **Move Up the Body**: Gradually work your way up through your legs, abdomen, arms, shoulders, and neck, tensing each muscle group for a few seconds and then relaxing.
- **Focus on Release**: As you release the tension in each muscle group, imagine letting go of the worries, stresses, or fears that are keeping you awake.
- **End with Deep Breathing**: Once you've relaxed all of your muscles, take a few deep breaths, focusing on the sensation of calm and peace in your body.

Creating a Peaceful Environment

Sometimes, physical changes to your environment can make a big difference in how easily you fall asleep. Consider these simple adjustments to help promote restful sleep:

- **Dim the lights** at least 30 minutes before bed to signal to your body that it's time to sleep.

- **Use calming scents** like lavender, chamomile, or frankincense to promote relaxation.

- **Turn off electronics** at least 30 minutes before bed. The blue light emitted by screens can disrupt your body's natural sleep-wake cycle.

Write in Your Gratitude Journal

Cultivating gratitude before bed is a great way to shift your focus away from what's keeping you awake and toward God's blessings. Each night, write down three things you are thankful for—this could be something that happened during the day, a personal accomplishment, or even the quiet peace of the night. This practice can help you end the day on a positive note, reducing feelings of frustration or anxiety that might contribute to insomnia.

Day 7
GOD'S PROMISE

Philippians 1:6 (NIV):
*"Being confident of this, that he who began a good work in you
will carry it on to completion until the day of Christ Jesus."*

As you continue your journey through these 31 days, you must remember that God is faithful to fulfill His promises, and this brings peace and confidence, leading to restful sleep. Philippians 1:6 reassures us that God is actively working in our lives, and His plans will come to fruition. His Word will never go void, and this will aid you in letting go of worry, fear, anxiety, or any demonic attack that seems to attempt to interrupt God's promise to you of sound sleep.

Imagine this: you put your head on the pillow tonight, and the world drops off your back. The anxieties, the tasks, the fantasies, the doubts are forgotten. Why? Because you are asleep in the invincible promise of God: He who started a good work in you will continue it. That is the sweet truth, isn't it?

This commitment is more than a few lines on a page. It's the bedrock of your stillness. It's the trust you have not because of what you can do but because of the One who has your future in His hands. No matter where you are in your walk with God, he never left you. His word has not changed. If you get discouraged, burned out, and don't know where to go next, know this: God is at work in you right now and He will finish it—when He is perfect and just when He is ready.

Keep in mind tonight as you shut your eyes, God's work in you isn't to make you perfect today. You have to believe that He is there for you, for His guidance, for His shaping every day. Sometimes it's slow and sometimes you feel stuck or at the crux of something. But don't despair, God doesn't give up on His mission. He finishes what He starts. Each struggle,

Unlock Deep Sleep Secrets

every tear, every cry...it is all for Him to use to get you into a better state of rest, of joy, and of purpose.

As Philippians 1:6 promises, God will "take it up to completion." What a relief! You don't need to worry about the future, or about being too good. God is good and He is doing the work on you day by day. Your life is an artist's studio. And God is always shaping you with His love and grace like an artist, taking time away from what is in front of Him to tweak, perfect, and apply the final touches.

So, while you are sleeping tonight, remember that your life is being made right by a loving Creator. You don't have to stress about the next and that you're not good enough. God tells you he will finish what he began. Your journey is under His watch, and He's on it.

This is the wonderful thing about God's promise: it does not give you hope for today only, but also hope for tonight as well. If you have faith in His word, you can sleep well at night, for God who has begun His work in you is not finished. And you are every day, the next day closer to His beautiful completeness.

Sleep well, tonight. God's got this. And He's got you.

Prayer for the Journey

Dear God, I approach Your throne of grace tonight, confident of the promise You gave in Philippians 1:6, **Being confident of this very thing, that he which hath begun a good work in you will perform it until the day of Jesus Christ:**

Lord, as Paul expresses his confidence in you, I too express my confidence in You. I am confident in your faithfulness to bring to completion, first of all, the work of salvation and spiritual growth You have started in my life. I am confident that even when life feels unfinished or uncertain, You are actively working on me. I thank you that the good work of becoming more like Jesus is not based on my efforts, but on Your faithfulness. I decree that my restful sleep is coming to completion in my life just as Jesus experienced restful sleep on the stormy seas.

Lord, I trust in Your perfect timing and process of restful sleep. I surrender my striving, and I choose to experience the peace that allows me to rest deeply tonight.

I declare I will sleep soundly; I have no worries, fears, concerns or panic attacks because I trust in Your divine promise of sleep. When I wake up, I will be refreshed and rejuvenated and will complete all my assigned tasks with excellence. I will rest on Your promises tonight. In Jesus' name. Amen.

31 Days to Overcoming Insomnia

JOURNAL

"Sound Sleep is Important"

Focus Verse Reflection
Begin by meditating on Philippians 1:6. As you wake up, remind yourself that God has begun a good work in you and will bring it to completion. Even though you may have faced challenges or anxieties, trust that God's purpose for your life is still unfolding, and He is present with you through every moment of your day.

Journaling Guided Reflections
How can I trust that God's work in me will continue today? What good work do I want to invite God into today?

_____
_____
_____
_____
_____
_____

Cognitive Renewal Statements

- I am confident that God is working in me, even when I don't see it. Today, I trust that He will bring His good work to completion, and I release all fears and doubts into His care.

Morning Mindful Rest Practices

Gratitude Stretch: Before getting out of bed, take a few moments to stretch slowly while thanking God for a new day. With each stretch, say something you're grateful for—this could be your health, family, your home, or just the simple gift of today. Gratitude helps shift your focus to God's goodness and sets a positive tone for the day ahead.

Afternoon Guided Reflections (Reflections & Preparing for Rest)

Focus Verse Reflection: As the day continues, reflect again on Philippians 1:6. Take a moment to pause, breathe deeply, and remember that God is actively at work in your life. No matter what has happened so far, He is faithful to complete His purpose in you.

Afternoon Cognitive Renewal Statements: God is working in me, and He will finish what He started. I am at peace, knowing that I don't have to do everything on my own. I rest in His promises.

Unlock Deep Sleep Secrets

> **Journaling Guided Reflections:** What worries or stresses have I been holding onto today? How can I surrender them to God, knowing He will continue His good work in me?

_____
_____
_____
_____

Evening Thoughts: Protecting Your Peace

Isaiah 32:18 is not just a promise about the physical peace of a home, but about developing an environment—internally and externally—that exhibits God's peace, protection, and rest. By protecting your home and heart, you are making space for God's presence to dwell richly in your life. Whether you're decluttering a space, practicing mindfulness, or releasing anxiety to God in prayer, every step you take toward a peaceful environment brings you closer to experiencing the fullness of His peace and security.

May your home, your heart, and your mind reflect God's care, peace, and rest, as you align your life with His promises of a secure and undisturbed place of rest.

Evening Mindful Rest Practices

> **Mindful Breathing with Scripture:** Set aside 5 minutes for a breathing exercise where you breathe deeply for a count of 4, hold for 4, and breathe out for 4. As you do, silently repeat the words from Philippians 1:6: "He who began a good work in me will bring it to completion." Let this truth sink in as you focus on your breath and feel God's peace settle in your heart.

Evening Guided Reflections (Preparing for Peaceful Sleep)

> **Focus Verse Reflection:** As the evening approaches, reflect once more on Philippians 1:6. Think about how God has been faithful to you throughout the day, whether you saw His work clearly or not. Trust that He is still at work, even while you sleep. There is nothing too small or too large for God to handle.
>
> ### *Journaling Guided Prompts*
> - What did I learn today about God's faithfulness?

_____
_____
_____
_____

31 Days to Overcoming Insomnia

- How can I leave my worries with God tonight, trusting that He is working even while I sleep?

_____
_____
_____
_____

Gratitude List
Create a list of things you are grateful for, particularly the ways you've seen God fulfill His promises in your life.

_____
_____
_____
_____

Bedtime Prayer
Develop a bedtime prayer that acknowledges God's promises and asks for peace as you sleep.

Reflection
After doing these things, pause and ask yourself:
- How do you feel about God's Word that He has placed in front of your heart?
- How can trusting that God will finish His work keep you awake at night?
- Take notes about what you notice or feel that you did not know before your reflections.

Weekly Theme
Day Review: Every seven days look back to Philippians 1:6 and consider the ministry God has accomplished for you. That might be through a journal, a prayer, even a ceremony of liturgy. Think of where you have come to, where you have been moving, where you still want God's work done. Thank God that He's still at work making you.

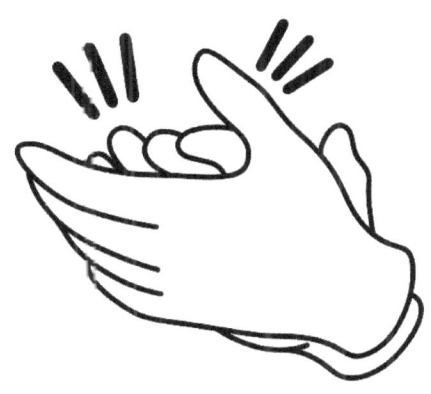

**WAY TO GO!!!
YOU MADE IT THROUGH
7 DAYS OF SLEEP REJUVENATION!**

Day 8
TRUSTING GOD'S WISDOM
OVER YOUR OWN UNDERSTANDING

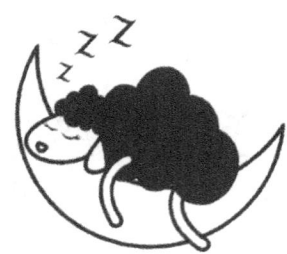

Proverbs 3:5-6 (NIV)
*"Trust in the Lord with all your heart and lean not on your own understanding;
in all your ways submit to him, and he will make your paths straight."*

Imagine this: it's a quiet, quiet night. Outside the window there's nothing happening, but inside your head is racing. The stakes in your choices, questions, and doubts are high. What if the road you are on is not the right one? What if the things you do aren't getting you where you want them to get you? You wish there were a map, an emphasis from the skies. If only you knew it would all work out for the best.

What if I showed you, though, that the absolute truth is going to revolutionize the way you sleep, the way you live, and the way you tackle all your challenges? So mighty that once you learn it, you won't have to go off on your own trying to figure it out. That is the reality: Choose God's wisdom rather than your own.

Proverbs 3:5-6 says this: "Follow the Lord with all your heart and turn not to your own knowledge; in all your ways give glory unto him, and he will make straight your paths." These verses aren't just tips — they're invitations to something bigger than human reason and reason itself. They're a call to give up your mind, to give up your anxieties, and to give up trying to run everything yourself. That's where it all gets peaceful.

And it happens to us all—we wrestle with ourselves. We eke it out, we ponder all the possibilities, and we take the best guesses we can. But here's the rub: We don't know very much. We have only what is before us. We can't know the future. We can't see the bigger picture. And for that reason, we can misunderstand. But God—God—sees it all. He notices the detours in your life you don't know how to take, the roadblocks you can't see coming,

Unlock Deep Sleep Secrets

and the lane that He has just laid out for you. And He can get you there even when you don't.

Imagine the freedom in that. And you don't have to know everything. And you don't need them all. So, you can no longer have to lug around the burden of wisdom on your shoulders, because God knows much more than we do. His script for you is so much more lovely, richer, spicier than anything you could have orchestrated. Once you put your full faith in Him, He leads—not with empty promises, but a real life-changing force.

Faith in God's knowledge is a leap of faith. It's the kind of trust that doesn't simply give God permission to take you somewhere; it gives up your will. It's giving your wants and your schedule to His plan. And the wonder is, if you believe in God that way, He doesn't just direct you; He plows you straight. He unblocks and lifts the clouds and brings you purpose, serenity, and happiness. That's the dream of a life where you're never out on your own and never out of your way.

And here's the best thing: this trust gives rest. You can sleep better when you place all your confidence in God's judgment. You can give up your dread, your terror, your doubt, and your unending effort. You will sleep easy because the Creator of the universe is directing you with knowledge that is far more superior to your own. You are in His hands. He's working it out on some level that you don't see right now, but you can believe it is made just for you.

So tonight when you close your eyes and go to sleep, give it up. Be in His hands, be it with your queries, concerns, choices. Let His wisdom takes over. You don't have to know it all. Confide in His infinite, infinite wisdom. When you do, you'll enter a silence unsurpassed in all understanding, a silence in which you can lie comfortably, knowing your way is being set on the right path, as you sleep.

God's wisdom over your understanding. That's trust, of the sort that shifts everything. It's the trust that frightens you and makes you happy and at ease and asleep. So, forget the responsibility of having to figure it all out on your own. Trust Him. And let Him take you to wherever beautiful you can imagine.

Goodnight, because you are walking in the counsel of Him Who carries the earth. He will make your paths straight. Trust in that promise.

Prayer for the Journey

Dear God, as I prepare to sleep tonight, I surrender my cares, my dreams and desires to You. Forgive me for relying on my own strength. I admit that, sometimes, I do try to cling to what I know and believe is best. But Your Word says in Proverbs 3:5-6 that I ought with all my heart to put my hope in Thee, and to depend not on my understanding. Yes Lord, I confess that there are many things I do not understand, and sometimes I try to carry

31 Days to Overcoming Insomnia

burdens that are too heavy for me. Tonight, I release those burdens into Your capable hands.

Lord, I acknowledge that You are wiser than me, therefore I place my cares into Your hands believing that You are leading me every step of the way even when I don't see it well. I acknowledge You in all my decisions, my family, my health and my future. Lord, I surrender control to You believing that Your ways and plans are far better than my own. I seek You earnestly in my decisions, actions and thoughts so that I can get clear direction and align myself with Your will. Thank you for Your peace and clarity that helps me overcome insomnia. I command my mind to be quiet and speak calmly over my spirit.

Thank you for being my shepherd and guide tonight. I lay all my hope and confidence in You and will not lean on my own understanding. I declare all my actions will be determined in accordance with Your word and not by me. I will trust You to sleep soundly without any warriors.

Thank You, Lord, for being my fortress, my protector, and my deliverer. I will continue to trust in You and will not rely on my own knowledge. In Jesus' name. Amen.

Unlock Deep Sleep Secrets

JOURNAL
"Sound Sleep is Important"

Morning: Surrendering the Day to God's Wisdom

Scripture Guided Reflection

Meditate on Proverbs 3:5-6. Acknowledge that your understanding is limited, but God's wisdom is infinite. Ask God to guide you today in ways that honor Him and lead you down paths of peace and righteousness.

Cognitive Renewal Statements

- I trust in the Lord with all my heart. Today, I choose not to lean on my own understanding, but to submit my ways to Him. I trust that He will guide me and make my paths straight.

Journaling Guided Reflections

What areas of my life do I need to surrender to God today? What areas am I tempted to rely on my own understanding instead of trusting God's wisdom?

_____
_____
_____
_____
_____
_____

Morning Mindful Rest Practices

Mindful Surrender: Begin your day with a moment of surrender. Sit quietly and close your eyes. Breathe deeply and release any worries or uncertainties to God. Say, *"Lord, I trust You with today. Guide my thoughts, decisions, and actions according to Your wisdom."* Let go of the need to control every situation and trust that God's guidance is sufficient.

Afternoon: Reaffirming Trust and Casting Your Worries

Scripture Reflection: Revisit 1 Peter 5:7 in the afternoon. Reflect on the idea of *casting your anxieties on God* because He cares for you. Take a moment to acknowledge any worries or burdens that are weighing you down, and trust that God is big enough to handle them.

31 Days to Overcoming Insomnia

Journaling Guided Reflections
What am I holding onto today that is causing me stress or anxiety? How can I intentionally release it to God, knowing He cares for me and is in control?

_____
_____
_____
_____
_____

Afternoon Cognitive Renewal Statements
- I cast all my anxieties on God, knowing that He cares for me. I do not have to carry these burdens alone. I trust in His wisdom to handle everything that concerns me.

Afternoon Mindful Rest Practices

Worry Box Exercise: Write down your worries or concerns on separate pieces of paper. As you write, prayerfully cast them onto God, saying, *"Lord, I surrender this concern to You. I trust Your wisdom to handle this better than I can."* Once written, put these papers in a box or envelope as a symbol of entrusting them to God. Leave the box in a place where you can "leave" your worries and mentally remind yourself that they are now in God's hands.

Evening: Reflecting on God's Guidance and Releasing Control

Scripture Reflection
As the evening approaches, reflect on the day and meditate on Proverbs 3:5-6 again. Did you trust God fully today, or did you find yourself relying on your own understanding in certain situations? Reflect on how God has guided you and thank Him for His wisdom and care.

_____
_____
_____
_____
_____

Journaling Guided Reflections
- Where did I experience God's wisdom today?

_____
_____
_____
_____
_____

Unlock Deep Sleep Secrets

- Were there moments when I relied on my own understanding?

  _____
  _____
  _____
  _____
  _____

- How can I seek God's guidance more fully tomorrow?

  _____
  _____
  _____
  _____
  _____

Evening Cognitive Renewal Statements

I release all the events of today into God's hands. I trust that His wisdom guided me, and I trust that He will continue to lead me. I rest in His care tonight, knowing He is working for my good.

Evening Mindful Rest Practices

- **Visualization of Surrender:** Before bed, imagine placing all your cares, choices, and troubles in God's hands. Picture yourself handing over your concerns to Him as though you were physically handing over an object. As you do this, say a prayer like, *"Lord, I trust You to work out everything I've surrendered to You. I trust that Your understanding is far greater than mine."* Allow yourself to feel a sense of peace knowing that you are not alone and that God is in control.

Day 9
SAFEGUARDING MY ENVIRONMENT

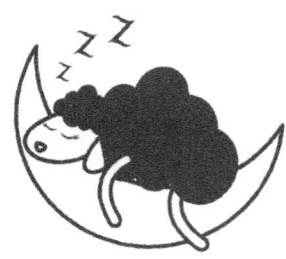

Isaiah 32:18 (NIV)
*"My people will live in peaceful dwelling places,
in secure homes, in undisturbed places of rest."*

Imagine this: A quiet, sleepless night. Outside, there is a hustle and bustle, but inside, your sanctuary is still. You're smelling good, your heart is in check, your mind is quiet. You are in a refuge, away from the hustle and bustle of the world. You have the feeling that the anxiety is lifted, and that there's something so reassuring about rest. That's the kind of silence you've been craving, and it's right there for you.

As Isaiah 32:18 shows us, life as God has it for His people is quite literally a beautiful thing: *My people will dwell in peace dwelling places, in safe houses, in steadfast places of rest.* And it is not some promise for the future – it is available to you now, in your life, in your space. But it takes an infusion. A change in the way you think about the world, how you secure it.

When we speak of "protecting" the environment, we are thinking about what we can do with physical things — lock doors, create walls, keep bad things out. But there is another protective layer we need to attend to: the psychological, mental, and spiritual space that we create all around us. Where we live, where we heart, where we brain, all these factors directly affect how well we can be able to find the home of tranquility God. Our living environment and emotional connection alongside cognitive processes determine our ability to find divine tranquility.

And this is the reality: Your space is not just your space; it's what you allow into your space. It comes from what you see, hear, think, and feel. And, as you would guard your physical house against threats, you must also guard your heart and mind against those

Unlock Deep Sleep Secrets

things that deny you tranquility. The noisy world outside can find its way inside, tumbling us with anxiety, fear, and stress. But God has a better way, and that's to be in "safe houses" and "peaceful places of refuge."

So how do we protect our environment and build these spaces of relaxation? Let's explore three powerful ways:

Guard Your Heart and Mind
What goes on in you shapes the outside. We are to "keep your heart, for all your works are made of it." Proverbs 4:23 says "your house will speak to your heart." If you live in a heart and mind full of negative energy, anxiety, and fear, then everything will become what is in your heart. But when you make the decision to live your heart in peace, love, and joy, you have a sanctuary where rest will grow. Guard your thoughts. Free your mind from turbulence, negative stories, icky friends, addictive behaviors. Swap them for something good for your soul: uplifting music, God's Word, positive thoughts, time in the woods.

Create a Physical Sanctuary
Your physical space should have peace in it. All the clutter, all the distraction, all the muck—everything contributes to your happiness. God wants you to live in "safe homes" – homes not only of your body, but of your mind and heart. Look around your space for a minute. Is it a place that gives you serenity? Or does it stress you out? Declutter, demystify, and unpack. Set up a sanctuary where you can be in a place where you feel at peace—through calm colors, smells, and peaceful spots where you can sit and think.

Guard Your Spiritual Environment
It is all based in your spiritual space. That's where you meet God, where you're energized, and where your safety is found. When you give room to God, you are giving room to God's peace. Keep a spiritual diary. Prayer, meditation, God's Word: Spend time with God. These rites protect your heart, putting you in the arms of God and He will give you rest. When you make your home and heart a rich, spiritual place, then only God can set you at peace.

The Result: Peaceful Dwelling Places
When you actively safeguard your environment—both the external and internal—you unlock the promise of Isaiah 32:18. God has designed you to live in *"peaceful dwelling places, in secure homes, in undisturbed places of rest."* This is His heart for you, and it's possible when you make the choice to protect what enters your life. Every decision, every action, every boundary you set creates a ripple effect that leads you to a more peaceful, restful life. As you prepare for sleep tonight, take a deep breath and reflect: **Is my environment a place of peace?** If there are areas of your heart, mind, or physical space that are filled with

31 Days to Overcoming Insomnia

clutter, stress, or unrest, it's time to take action. Guard your environment like the precious sanctuary it is and watch as God's peace begins to fill every corner of your life.
God's promise of peace is not just a future hope; it's a present reality. He's calling you to live in secure homes, to rest in undisturbed places, and to experience the kind of peace that the world cannot offer. Safeguard your environment, and in doing so, you will find yourself resting in God's perfect peace, tonight and every night.

So tonight, as you lay down to sleep, let the stillness of your environment remind you of God's perfect rest. Close your eyes knowing that you've done your part to protect your heart, your home, and your soul. You are safe. You are secure. And you are at peace.

Prayer for the Journey

Dear God, as I lie down, I bow before You with my heart filled with thankfulness for the way You have kept me alive. Thank you for the comfort that only Your word can provide. I am really grateful for the promises that You have made in Your word. You promised in Isaiah 32:18 that **"my people shall dwell in a peaceable habitation, and in sure dwellings, and in quiet resting places."** *Based on this verse, I decree that I have received Your promise of* **peaceable habitation**; *which is, freedom from all chaos in the world that hinders my sweet sleep and a life of stability.*

I decree that I **remain in sure dwellings,** *which emphasizes the certainty and security found in Your presence. I decree that I* **dwell in quiet resting places**, *which suggests the calm that fills my heart because I trust in You for help to fight for sweet sleep. Lord Jesus, thanks for Your peace that will help me transcend circumstances and bring restful sleep even in turbulent times.*

Thank you for emphasizing Your desire to ensure a stable and tranquil environment for me. Your promise of divine protection and serenity shows Your heart to provide not just physical safety but inner peace and assurance; which does well for sweet sleep.

Once again, thank you for Your promise of peace and security. Let Your angel guard my house, my family, and everything I hold dear. Lord, thank you for protecting my home from turmoil and creating and making it a place of serenity. Because You reign in my house, I know that I will be kept safe and sound at night as I sleep. I decree that my house is a haven of peace and is in God's protection. No weapon formed against me shall succeed because I'm under God's protection. Tonight, I decree that I will be granted sleep in tranquility, I turn over all my worries to You and know that You are watching over my world in the mighty name of Jesus. Amen.   (And that's exactly how it will be!)

Unlock Deep Sleep Secrets

JOURNAL
"Sound Sleep is Important"

Morning Cognitive Renewal Statements
I am grateful for the peace God has promised me. As I begin this day, I choose to live in harmony with His plan. My home is a place of security and rest, where God's presence dwells.

Morning Journal Guided Reflections

What steps can I take today to create peace in my environment?
_____
_____
_____
_____
_____
_____
_____
_____

How can I be intentional about guarding my home and my heart from stress, conflict, or distractions?
_____
_____
_____
_____
_____
_____
_____
_____

This prompt above should inspire you to think about how you can actively adopt a peaceful environment at the start of the day. What are the easy ways you can prepare your home—physically, emotionally, and spiritually—to reflect God's peace?

Morning Mindful Rest Practices: Declutter and Clear Space

Activity
Declutter a Space in Your Home: Choose a small area of your home—perhaps your desk, a closet, or your kitchen counter—and clear out anything that's causing stress, clutter, or distraction. As you do, invite God's peace into that space, saying a prayer like, *"Lord, I*

31 Days to Overcoming Insomnia

thank You for this space, and I invite Your peace to fill it. May this space reflect Your presence in my life."

Purpose
Physical clutter can often mirror emotional or mental clutter. By clearing space, you are physically and symbolically making room for peace, rest, and order. It also sets the tone for how you will care for the rest of your environment.

Afternoon Cognitive Renewal Statement

Cognitive Renewal Statement

- As I move through this day, I choose peace over anxiety. I trust that God is my protector, and I am safe in His care. My mind, heart, and surroundings are secure.

Purpose: Letting Go of Stress and Fostering Calm

- This affirmation helps to refocus your energy on God's security and protection. It serves as a reminder that you do not need to carry the burden of worry; your environment—both physical and emotional—is safe in God's hands.

Afternoon Journal Guided Reflections

What worries or stresses from the day have disturbed my peace so far?

_____
_____
_____

How can I release these things to God and reclaim my environment for peace and rest?

_____
_____
_____

Reflection
Take a few minutes to reflect on the sources of stress or anxiety in your day so far. Write down any thoughts or concerns that are keeping you from feeling at peace. Afterward, release them to God in prayer and ask for His peace to restore you.

_____
_____
_____
_____

Unlock Deep Sleep Secrets

Afternoon Mindful Rest Practices: Mindful Prayer and Breathing

Activity
Mindful Breathing and Prayer: Sit quietly for five minutes and breathe deeply. As you breathe in, pray, *"Lord, fill me with Your peace."* As you breathe out, pray, *"I release my anxieties and worries into Your hands."* Repeat this process for several minutes to restore your heart and mind.

Purpose
Mindful breathing is a practice that calms the nervous system, reduces stress, and helps reset the body. Coupled with prayer, it becomes a powerful tool for safeguarding your emotional environment by focusing on God's peace and letting go of any worries.

Evening Affirmation: Surrendering the Day and Embracing Peaceful Rest

Cognitive Renewal Statements

- I surrender all my worries and cares to God. As I lay down to sleep tonight, I trust in His protection and peace. My home is a sanctuary of rest, and I receive the peaceful sleep God promises.

Purpose

- This affirmation helps you mentally release the stresses of the day and invite God's protection over your home and heart. It reminds you that peace is available, and you can rest secure in God's care.

Evening Journal Guided Reflections

What emotions or worries am I holding onto from today?

_____
_____
_____
_____

How can I intentionally release these as I prepare for rest tonight?

_____
_____
_____
_____

31 Days to Overcoming Insomnia

Reflection

Reflect on your emotional state as you prepare for bed. Write anything that may still be weighing on your mind. Afterward, ask God to help you release these things, trusting that He will care for them as you rest.

_____
_____
_____
_____
_____

Evening Mindful Rest Practices: Create a Calming Bedtime Ritual

Activity - Create a Restful Routine

Begin a calming bedtime ritual to help you transition from the busyness of the day to a peaceful night's rest. This might include activities like dimming the lights, reading a devotional or Scripture, listening to calming music or nature sounds, or practicing deep breathing.

Purpose

A calming routine helps to prepare your body and mind for rest, signaling that it's time to wind down. This reinforces the idea of your environment being a place of peace and rest, aligning with God's desire for you to have "undisturbed places of rest" (Isaiah 32:18).

Weekly Guided Reflection: Safeguarding My Environment for Peace and Rest

At the end of each week, take time to reflect on your journey toward safeguarding your environment. Use the following questions to guide your reflection:

Reflection Prompt: How have I been able to create a peaceful environment this week? What practices or changes have helped me experience more security and rest? What areas still need attention or improvement in my emotional or physical environment?

_____
_____
_____
_____
_____
_____
_____
_____

Unlock Deep Sleep Secrets

Scripture Reflection
"My people will live in peaceful dwelling places, in secure homes, in undisturbed places of rest." — Isaiah 32:18

Reflect on how you've experienced God's promise of peace this week. In what ways have you created a more peaceful home, both physically and emotionally?

_____
_____
_____
_____
_____

How can you continue to safeguard your environment moving forward?

_____
_____
_____
_____
_____

Day 10
CHRIST PROVIDES YOU WITH THE STRENGTH YOU NEED

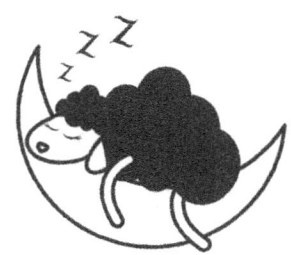

Isaiah 40:29-31 (NIV)
*"He gives strength to the weary and increases the power of the weak
... those who hope in the Lord will renew their strength."*

Philippians 4:13 KJV
"I can do all things through Christ which strengtheneth me."

It Is the Hidden Power Behind Unbridled Power

Has anything ever been so consuming that your body, your mind, and your soul were empty? Maybe it's the struggle, maybe it's the night of worry, or it's the stress of life just building up. You're exhausted. Tired. Weary beyond measure. You seek power all around you, but not certain it's going to be enough.

But the reality is: Christ gives you strength when you don't have it, because He can give you strength when no one else can.

Consider that for a moment. Christ, the Creator of all things, the glue-maker, the King of Kings, gives you His power to get through it all. And when you draw from His power, something wonderful happens: You will fly.

The Promise of Unfailing Strength

In Isaiah 40:29-31 is one of the most beautiful promises of all Scripture. It begins with the universally human condition of fatigue and exhaustion: *"He strengthens the tired and magnifies the weak."* How many of us can get over that? We push, we fight, we try, but sometimes it's too much. We can't stop fighting and we lose energy. Even children get tired

Unlock Deep Sleep Secrets

and worn out. Even the best individuals can get tired. Even the unstoppable can overheat. And this is where God's promise gets funny. For they who trust in the Lord, the fatigued will be restored. You don't have to keep trying. If you hope and believe on Christ, He will resurrect you. And not a trace—He will revive you so abundantly that you'll feel as if you're on eagle wings.

Can you picture it? Humming on eagle wings, running and not tired, walking and not fainting. This is not about a quick energy fix. It's getting divine, supernatural power that gets you where you never could have imagined. When you are too tired to go on, God fills you with a power that you cannot resist.

The Strength of Christ in You
This is the power of God; the Apostle Paul enjoins us in Philippians 4:13: *"I can do all things through him who gives me strength."* Not from self-reliance, but because we know Christ's power. Not to get up by your bootstraps and claw your way out of it. That's letting Christ have your weakness and letting Him work through you.

See, when you are linked to Christ, your vulnerability is a place where His power can show up. This is not about you; this is about Christ in you and through you. If it is something you have to do, if you're tired or just don't have the time to keep up with your life, Christ says, "I got you. Lean on Me. I'll help you fight."

Strength That Soars
We have Isaiah 40:31, the glorious vision of flying on wings like eagles. Eagles fly with ease through the air, on the winds, to fantastic heights, and without raising their wings. That's the power that God says He will give you. It's the muscle that keeps you above your troubles, over your fatigue, above your setbacks.

With Christ on your side, you don't survive; you thrive. And you'll get further, faster and easier than you ever could have imagined. You will have calm in the middle of the storm. You will walk with courage in the midst of the trouble of life, by the grace of Him, and not faint in the sight of Him. His strength doesn't make you get through the day – it makes you who is bigger than you thought you could be. His strength transforms you into someone much stronger than you previously thought possible.

Christ's Strength for Your Sleep
Suppose you apply this truth to your sleep. Tonight, when you go to sleep, you know Christ is providing you with the power. Even when you are most defeated, when you have nowhere to go but down, His power can lift you into sweet sleep.

If you trust in Christ, your rest becomes more than just physical rest, but a time to tap into His healing hand. Your soul needs the renewing hand of Christ. He yields that in Him, you

31 Days to Overcoming Insomnia

shall rest, be strong, and be at peace. Christ will be regenerating you as you lie down, re-getting you up for the day.

When you wake up, you won't need to be self-sufficient to get through it. The power of Christ will be with you and you will go above the obstacles, running endurance and walking content. His power is ever-present, always available, never-enough.

The Invitation to Trust

But what does this mean for you now? It is an invitation for you to put your weak points in Christ's hands and let Him bolster you. It's about believing that He is enough to see you through the darkest days, the darkest moments, the darkest chastening. You don't have to do the work alone. Christ is giving it to you to hold and He will be able to help you through.

Tonight, when you fall asleep, breathe in deeply and let go of everything that's holding you back. Remember that Christ is your power. He is regenerating you, healing you, re-setting you up for whatever's next. You will wake with His power–fly like an eagle, run not tiring out, walk without falling down.

Christ gives you the power. Rest in His power. Sleep deeply in His care and wake up to His unlimited power for your life.

Prayer for the Journey

*Dear God, it's been 10 days since I began trusting you for my sound sleep. The number 10 signifies **completeness, divine order, and the perfection of your will**. I decree that restful sleep for me is coming to completion, it's your divine order that the night was given to rest and I accept your perfect will for sweet sleep for me tonight. Thank you for the promise you made in Isaiah chapter 40 verses 29 to 31. This text reminds me of your dominion, strength and compassion. Lord, you dominate, you're all powerful and compassionate. Look upon me with compassion tonight as I prepare for restful sleep. Show me how to overcome the challenges that hinder me from getting good sleep. Give me the strength to power through the thoughts that hinder me from getting good sleep. Look upon me with compassion. I have messed up and so I acknowledge the weariness and the burdens I carry.*

Lord as your word promises, help me mount up on wings as eagles, give me the divine enablement and the capacity to rise above the challenges that leave me in state of sleeplessness, as I wait on you for direction.

Lord, you know no matter how strong or how young, everyone grows weary at some point. The key is waiting on you and that's exactly what I am doing. Lord, I hopefully expect you to restore my sleep, I trust and rely on you. Even in the face of this challenge of insomnia, I still believe your power is limitless and accessible to help bring me through.

Unlock Deep Sleep Secrets

Your resources are inexhaustible, and I rest in your renewing power. Lord, I decree that I am replenished and sustained by you, enabling me to face challenges with renewed vigor.

Lord Jesus as I prepare for rest. I thank you again, for the strength which you have already given me. Thank you for your continuous strength throughout the journey! When I feel like giving up, I will remember Your word and trust You for your security. I will Not lean on my ideas but will put my trust in you.

I decree You are my strength, You are my mind regulator. I decree I have the mind of Christ and therefore, no negative thought, lingering thoughts, emotions will interfere with my sleep.

You are my refuge and my strength, Lord. "I trust that You are giving me all the strength I could ever ask for now and tomorrow. I rely on Your infinite love and strength. In Jesus' name, Amen.

31 Days to Overcoming Insomnia

JOURNAL

"Sound Sleep is Important"

Morning Cognitive Renewal Statements

- Today, I trust in Christ to give me the strength I need for whatever comes my way.
- I am not alone in my struggles—God is with me, and His strength is made perfect in my weakness.
- I can do all things through Christ who strengthens me, including facing challenges today with peace.
- I wait upon the Lord, and He will renew my strength. I am equipped for today.
- With Christ's help, I will run without weariness and walk without fainting.

Morning Guided Reflections

- Begin your day with a quiet moment to reflect on Isaiah 40:29-31 and Philippians 4:13. Close your eyes and breathe deeply, envisioning yourself standing strong in Christ's power.
- As you breathe in, say, "I receive strength from Christ."
- As you breathe out, say, "I let go of all worries and rest in His peace."

Evening Cognitive Renewal Statements

- I rest in the strength of the Lord. He is my refuge and my source of peace.
- I trust that God is in control of my circumstances, and I surrender my worries to Him tonight.
- Christ's strength empowers me to sleep soundly and peacefully. I let go of all burdens.
- I am surrounded by God's love, and I trust that He is renewing me even as I sleep.
- As I wait upon the Lord, He renews my strength. I trust that I will wake up refreshed tomorrow.

Evening Guided Reflections

- Before you settle into bed, take a moment to reflect on your day.
- Ask yourself, "Where did I need Christ's strength today? How did He sustain me?"
- Picture yourself releasing all the stresses and burdens from the day into God's hands.

Unlock Deep Sleep Secrets

- Spend a few minutes in prayer, asking for God's peace to fill your heart and mind as you prepare to rest.

Sleep Guided Reflections and Journaling
Before Bed (to encourage trust and peace):

What worries or stresses am I carrying that I need to surrender to Christ tonight?

_____
_____
_____
_____
_____

How has God strengthened me today? Even in my weaknesses, I can see His power at work.

_____
_____
_____
_____

Write down any thoughts or worries in your journal, then pray over them, asking Christ to take them from you and give you His peace instead.

_____
_____
_____
_____

After Waking (to reinforce Christ's strength)

How did I experience God's strength while I was sleeping?

_____
_____
_____
_____

Did I feel His peace throughout the night?

_____
_____
_____
_____

31 Days to Overcoming Insomnia

Write about how you feel after waking up. Are you more at peace with yourself? More hopeful? Ask God to help you trust in His strength for the day ahead.

_____
_____
_____
_____

Mindful Rest Practices for Restful Sleep

- **Scripture Meditation:**
    - Take 5-10 minutes before sleep to meditate on Isaiah 40:29-31 and Philippians 4:13.
    - Close your eyes and repeat each verse softly in your mind. Allow the words to sink in deeply.
    - Visualize yourself soaring on wings like eagles—light, free, and strong in Christ.

- **Progressive Muscle Relaxation (PRM):**
    - As you prepare to sleep, do a body scan starting at your toes and working your way up.
    - Tighten and then relax each muscle group as you breathe deeply.
    - As you do this, remind yourself, *"Christ is the source of my strength; I let go of tension and rest in His peace."*

- **Breathing Exercise:**
    - Try the 4-7-8 breathing technique to calm your nervous system:
        - Inhale deeply through your nose for a count of 4.
        - Hold the breath for a count of 7.
        - Exhale slowly through your mouth for a count of 8.
        - Repeat for 3-4 cycles, focusing on releasing all anxiety and trusting God's strength to carry you into a peaceful sleep.

- **Nightly Prayer**
    - **(Surrender and Trust):** As you prepare to sleep tonight, whisper a prayer in the quiet of the night.
    - *"Dear God, I offer up my concerns and fears to You, along with my weariness. Thank you for being my source of strength. I have faith in Your ability to grant me peace for my body and soul. May I arise refreshed and prepared to face tomorrow with Your guidance. Amen."*

Day 11
MORNING MENTAL CLARITY

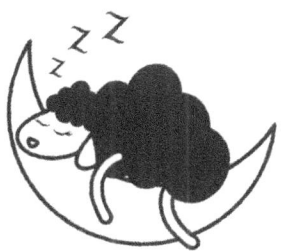

Proverbs 3:5-6 (NIV):
"Trust in the Lord with all your heart and lean not on your own understanding; in all your ways submit to him, and he will make your paths straight."

Waking Up with A Purpose and Joy
It's early morning outside your window, and the wind knocks you awake from the night. But your head goes aflutter before you even get out of bed. The to-do list, the tattletales, the list of agendas, they're already filling your head. Is your morning a mad dash, or do you wake up spry, ready to take on the day with intention?

A secret: Getting out of bed in the morning starts with trust. When you awake and give God the reins of your day, it's a wonder: you have thoughts that go according to His peace. And clarity doesn't come from trying to understand it all on your own; it comes from believing God is going to take you wherever you go.

The Power of Trust
There's a rich teaching in Proverbs 3:5-6 that will make mornings so much clearer: "Lean not on your own understanding, but in the Lord." We awake thinking that all of the answers to our problems, all of the answers to our problems are located somewhere in our own heads. But the reality is that we know little of what's happening and can get lost in our own jumbled thinking and fear of being unknowable.

But when we believe God, when we let go of wanting to have the finger on all the levers, He clears the mist and brings us to the straight. If we trust God, we don't need to see with a pedantic lens. Instead, we can count on His wisdom, His guidance, and His stillness to carry us throughout the day.

31 Days to Overcoming Insomnia

The New Way to Start Your Day with You
And suppose you wake up feeling like you have the answer, not that you've got it all figured out, but because you gave up your plans to the Master of Perspective. No more do you have to bear all the clutter in your head—you can leave it with God. Here's how you can start:

> ***Get Up and Take a Breath:*** Before you climb out of bed and send your mind on an exhilarating tour of anxieties and to-dos, stop and breathe in. Settle your mind. No longer do you need to make it all about you. But don't be afraid. God will show you the way.
>
> ***Be Committed to God:*** Proverbs 3:6 *"In all your ways submit to him, and he will make your paths straight."* Commit your day to God. Ask Him for guidance. Work day, sleep day, or day of doubt: Give your plans to Him. Just know that He will make decisions and you will do things and think things.
>
> ***Let God Be in Charge:*** If you believe in God, then you believe God is in charge. He'll straighten out your brain clutter and bring your paths to square one. You don't have to figure it all out in your head right now; let God guide you. When you are dependent on Him, in the face of doubt, you will rest.
>
> ***His Peace:*** While you are doing your morning walk, think of peace. And if anxiety is starting to get in, remember to come back to faith. Read out loud the scripture: "Fear the Lord with all your heart." Let the reality of God come over you. His serenity will be there for your heart and your mind, and you'll have clarity in the midst of it all.

The Product of Trust: Clear Directions to Come
What is nice about having faith in God is that He doesn't leave you lost in the fog. He says He'll put your tracks straight. That way you can go through the day with peace of mind, clarity, and meaning. Now you won't have to fumble through the muddle of your own thoughts but instead, walk the course that He has laid before you with confidence, stillness, and safety.

When you lay down your plans before Him, you'll start to automatically do His will. Choices will be easier. All the huffing and puffing will lift, and you'll see God's hand on your life more clearly. Having all the answers is not the secret of morning clarity–it is putting your trust in the Master.

Putting Your Beliefs to the Test for the Rest of Your Life
Do not forget that your brain is not finished once you're out of bed. You will still believe the Lord with all your heart today when you confront the day. Continue giving up your mind, your thoughts, and your agenda to Him. Whenever you make a choice, whether large or small, know that He is with you, making you straight.

Unlock Deep Sleep Secrets

The next time your brain gets bogged down and the clutter starts to re-infest, take a deep breath and point back to Proverbs 3:5-6. Keep your eyes on the Lord and He will help you to see. You'll live your day with Him in the background, so you can experience it with meaning and hope.

A Powerful Start

So next time you lie down this evening, remember that the basis for mental clarity is trust. If you give God 100% of your head, your day, and your decisions, He will open up the cloud of your thoughts and get you straight. You will sleep soundly knowing that, when you rise tomorrow, you will have all the lucidity and calmness only God can bring.

Confide in Him and start your day with a clear head and a calm heart. Faith in God is the very beginning of your day's mental clarity, believe it first thing in the morning.

Prayer for the Journey

Dear God, as I prepare for bed, I want to thank you for how You held my hand today. I want to thank you in advance for the sound sleep tonight. You know how my mind was bombarded with thoughts and now I give them to You. Thank you for bringing into remembrance Philippians 4:7 that Your peace surpasses all understanding and will you guard my heart and mind in Christ Jesus and Proverbs 3:5-6, "Trust in the Lord with all your heart and lean not on your own understanding; in all your ways submit to Him, and He will make your paths straight."

Lord, I understand I can't live a peaceful life without You, so I surrender all those thoughts that have been bombarding my mind to You. I forgive myself for not trusting You. Now Lord, I release all my worry, thoughts, hurts, and anxiety to You. I need You to declutter my mind, so I can obtain rest and wake up rejuvenated.

Lord, thank You for peace, clarity of mind, and a good night's sleep. I give You my mind and my life, and I am sure that you'll do everything for me. In Jesus' name. Amen.

31 Days to Overcoming Insomnia

JOURNAL
"Sound Sleep is Important"

Morning Cognitive Renewal Statements

- Today, I trust in God's wisdom and guidance. My mind is clear, and I am filled with peace.

Begin your day by repeating this affirmation aloud or silently as you get ready. By speaking these words, you set a positive intention for mental clarity and reliance on God.

Morning Journal Guided Reflections

How do you typically feel when you wake up in the morning? Reflect on any thoughts or worries that often cloud your mind.

_____
_____
_____
_____
_____
_____

How can you start your day by trusting in God's wisdom instead of your own understanding?

_____
_____
_____
_____
_____
_____

Write a prayer, asking God to renew your mind each morning and provide you with mental clarity and peace for the day ahead.

_____
_____
_____
_____
_____
_____
_____

Unlock Deep Sleep Secrets

Morning Mindful Rest Practices for Mental Clarity

Scripture Meditation
- Before starting your day, spend a few minutes meditating on a verse like Proverbs 3:5-6 or Romans 12:2. As you reflect, ask God to clear away any mental clutter and guide your thoughts for the day. You can sit quietly and repeat the verse or write it down in your journal as a form of meditation.

Mindful Breathing Exercise
- Practice a deep breathing exercise to center your mind and release any tension. Inhale deeply for 4 seconds, hold for 4 seconds, and exhale slowly for 6 seconds. While you breathe, focus on a calming phrase like "God clears my mind" or "I trust in God's guidance."

Morning Gratitude Reflection
- As soon as you wake up, list three things you are thankful for. By starting the day with gratitude, you shift your focus from worries or stress to God's blessings, which promotes mental clarity and peace.

_____
_____
_____
_____
_____

Prayer Walk
Go for a brief morning walk while praying or reflecting on scripture. Being outside in nature can help refresh your mind and bring clarity. As you walk, focus on the sounds around you and let the natural beauty help you reconnect with God.

Brain-Dump Journaling
Before diving into your day's tasks, spend a few minutes writing down everything on your mind, both good and bad. This exercise helps clear mental clutter, so you can focus on what's truly important. After writing, ask God to give you peace and guidance for the day.

_____
_____
_____
_____
_____
_____

31 Days to Overcoming Insomnia

Evening Cognitive Renewal Statements

- I rest; I release my worries to God. He renews my mind and brings clarity and peace for tomorrow.

Repeat this affirmation before bed, allowing it to calm your mind and prepare you for a restful night. Trust that God will refresh you as you sleep, giving you the strength and clarity you need for the next day.

Evening Mindful Rest Practices to Wind Down for Restful Sleep

Mental clarity during the day sets the stage for a peaceful evening and restful sleep. These activities help ease the transition from a busy day to a calm, centered night.

- **Evening Reflection and Prayer**
  Before going to bed, reflect on how you spent your day. Were you able to maintain clarity and peace? Pray for guidance and release, asking God to clear your mind of any lingering stress or worries. Surrender everything into His care.

- **Mindful Journaling**
  Write a short entry in your sleep journal. This can include thoughts about your day, any challenges you faced, or things you are grateful for. Reflect on how God helped you through the day and express your gratitude for His presence. This practice helps to clear your mind before sleep.

Day 12
HIS SPIRIT DWELLS IN YOU

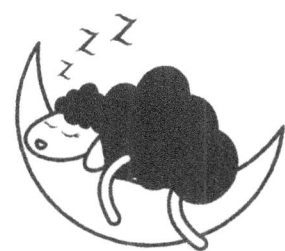

Romans 8:11 (NIV):
"And if the Spirit of him who raised Jesus from the dead is living in you, he who raised Christ from the dead will also give life to your mortal bodies because of his Spirit who lives in you."

When it comes to finding rest—both physically and spiritually—there is great comfort in knowing that God's Spirit dwells within us. This truth is a source of strength, peace, and renewal. In Romans 8:11, we are reminded that the same Spirit who raised Jesus from the dead lives in us, giving life and vitality to our bodies and minds. Understanding and embracing this truth can help us experience deeper rest and peace, knowing that God's Spirit is always present, even during times of restlessness or anxiety. Because Jesus's spirit lives inside of you, there must be some change. That change which takes place from inside will manifest from the outside, which will cause you to talk right, walk right, and have an attitude adjustment in your thinking.

Scriptural Reflection
Romans 8:11 (NIV): *"And if the Spirit of him who raised Jesus from the dead is living in you, he who raised Christ from the dead will also give life to your mortal bodies because of his Spirit who lives in you."*

This verse is a reminder of the profound gift of God's presence within us. The Holy Spirit, the same Spirit that raised Jesus from the dead, now dwells in every believer. This indwelling of the Holy Spirit provides us with strength, peace, and comfort, and it plays a key role in transforming our lives to reflect God's love and truth. It's also foundational in our journey toward inner peace, mental clarity, and a restful night's sleep.

31 Days to Overcoming Insomnia

Understanding that **God's Spirit dwells in you** means that His power, comfort, guidance, and presence are always available to you. This reality can bring great peace, especially when you need assurance that you are never alone, you are empowered to live a godly life, and your body and soul are being renewed by the Spirit. It reminds you that no matter the challenges you face, God's Spirit is at work within you, providing what you need.

How Does God's Spirit Dwell in You?

- *Indwelling through the Holy Spirit*
  The Holy Spirit is a gift to all who believe. It is the Holy Spirit that lives inside you when you accept Jesus Christ as your Savior. This is a spiritual truth that goes beyond thoughts and feelings. He is in you whether you "feel" His presence or not. You can live according to God's will with the help of the Spirit, who leads you in the truth and gives you the tools you need for every good work.

- *Guidance and Comfort*
  The Holy Spirit guides us by convicting our minds, teaching us God's truth, and giving us comfort when we're going through hard times. The Holy Spirit brings peace, clarity, and direction when you are feeling stressed, anxious, or lost. When the Holy Spirit is with you, it brings peace that goes beyond understanding. It helps you calm down and make decisions.

- *Empowerment and Strength*
  God's Spirit empowers you to live a triumphant life, free from the oppression of sin and fear. The Spirit strengthens you in your weakness, qualifying you to persevere through difficulties and remain steadfast in faith. When you feel inadequate or overwhelmed, the Holy Spirit within you is a constant source of strength.

- *Renewal of Mind and Body*
  Romans 8:11 speaks of the Spirit giving life to your mortal body. This renewal extends beyond just your spiritual state—it also brings healing and restoration to your physical and emotional well-being. The indwelling Spirit works in you to heal brokenness, renew your mind, and give peace to your soul, ultimately contributing to sound, restful sleep

Prayer for the Journey
Dear God, I ask that You let Your Spirit fill me, to quiet my heart and mind, to give me a deep peace as I get ready to sleep. And let Your presence surround me, and Your Spirit of Life renew my body, mind and heart. I trust that Your Spirit would be in me while I rest, regenerating my strength, regenerating my spirit.

Unlock Deep Sleep Secrets

Jesus I am aware that Your Spirit heals, calms and rests and declares that as Your Spirit dwells in me, I will sleep well and rise refreshed. I give away every worry and burden, knowing that You are there for me, safeguarding me, and sustaining me with breath and rest.

I decree and declare that the Spirit of God fills me with peace, rest, and renewal. I will lie down in peace because the Holy Spirit is giving life to my flesh and to my spirit. Today, I decree that the Spirit who raised Christ from the dead fills me with divine tranquility and strength. I am in the care and protection of God's Spirit and will be awakened, clean, and restored.

Thank you Lord for Your Spirit that dwells in me, that enables me with strength and peace to walk in Your defined order. I trust Your presence, and I lie down under Your shadow tonight. In Jesus' name. Amen.

31 Days to Overcoming Insomnia

JOURNAL

"Sound Sleep is Important"

Morning Cognitive Renewal Statements

- The Holy Spirit dwells within me, bringing life and peace to my body and mind. I am renewed by His presence. I have all the strength I need to face today.

Begin each morning by speaking this affirmation aloud or silently as you prepare for the day. Let these words remind you of the powerful presence of the Holy Spirit within you, guiding you throughout the day.

Morning Guided Reflections for Reflecting on God's Spirit in You

Acknowledge His Presence
Begin your day by acknowledging that the Holy Spirit is within you. Take a moment to consciously invite God's Spirit to lead you today. Reflect on the power and peace that comes from knowing that His presence dwells in you.

Prompt: "Holy Spirit, I thank You for dwelling within me. Guide me, empower me, and give me peace as I begin this day."

Prayer for Empowerment
Ask the Holy Spirit to empower you for the day ahead. Whether it's a challenging task at work, a difficult conversation, or a personal struggle, invite the Spirit to give you strength and wisdom.

Prompt: "Holy Spirit, empower me today. Fill me with Your strength and peace and guide me in all I do."

Journal Guided Reflections
Reflect on the significance of the Holy Spirit living within you. How does this truth affect how you approach moments of stress, restlessness, or anxiety?

_____
_____
_____
_____
_____

Unlock Deep Sleep Secrets

When you feel weary, how can you remind yourself that God's Spirit dwells within you, offering renewal and peace?

_____
_____
_____
_____

Write a prayer inviting the Holy Spirit to bring you peace and clarity as you rest, and to remind you of His presence in your daily life.

_____
_____
_____
_____
_____

Morning Mindful Rest Practices for Renewing with the Spirit

Morning Breath Prayer

- Begin your day by centering yourself through deep breathing.
- As you inhale, silently pray, "Holy Spirit, fill me."
- As you exhale, pray, "Bring life to my body and mind."
- Repeat this for several minutes, inviting the Holy Spirit to refresh and guide you for the day ahead.

Morning Scripture Meditation

Read today's daily scripture Romans 8:11 each morning. Reflect on the truth that the same Spirit who raised Christ from the dead is living in you. Meditate on the power and peace this brings, allowing it to set a foundation for your day. Consider writing the verse on a note to carry with you or display in a visible place as a reminder.

Spirit-Led Journaling

Before you begin your daily activities, write in your journal about the areas of your life where you need the Holy Spirit's guidance, strength, or peace. Ask the Holy Spirit to dwell richly in those areas and to provide you with the clarity, rest, and wisdom you need.

_____
_____
_____
_____
_____

31 Days to Overcoming Insomnia

Gratitude and Presence Walk
Take a brief walk in the morning, either outside or in a peaceful space, and focus on the presence of the Holy Spirit within you. As you walk, express gratitude for the Spirit's indwelling and for the life and strength He brings you. Notice the sensations around you and let them serve as reminders of God's life-giving Spirit at work within you.

Afternoon Guided Reflections to Stay Connected to His Spirit

Affirmation of His Empowering Presence
Throughout the afternoon, remind yourself of the empowering presence of the Holy Spirit within you.

Midday Check-In
Take a few minutes during the afternoon to check in with yourself. Reflect on how you've felt the Holy Spirit guiding or empowering you during the day. If you've felt stressed or distracted, use this time to reconnect and ask for renewed peace and clarity. *Prompt*: "Holy Spirit, I need Your peace and guidance as I continue my day. Renew my heart and mind with Your presence."

Breathing Exercise for Peace
Practice a simple breathing exercise to invite calmness and clarity. Breathe in deeply, imagining the Holy Spirit filling you with peace and breathe out any stress or worry. *Prompt*: "As I breathe in, I welcome Your peace, Holy Spirit. As I breathe out, I release all that is weighing on me."

Evening Mindful Rest Practices for Rest in the Spirit

Evening Cognitive Renewal Statements
The Spirit of God lives in me, renewing my mind and body as I rest. I release my worries, trusting in His peace and presence.

Repeat this affirmation before bed as a way to release any lingering stress or anxiety, trusting that the Holy Spirit will renew you as you sleep. Let these words comfort you, knowing that God's Spirit is always with you.

Evening Reflection and Prayer
Before bed, take a few moments to reflect on how the Holy Spirit has guided you throughout the day. Journal about moments when you felt His presence and how He helped you find peace or strength. End your reflection with a prayer, inviting the Holy Spirit to give you rest and renewal for the night.

Unlock Deep Sleep Secrets

Progressive Relaxation with the Spirit
As you prepare for sleep, practice progressive muscle relaxation, tense and releasing each muscle group from your toes to your head. As you do this, silently invite the Holy Spirit into your body, praying, *"Holy Spirit, bring peace to my body and mind."* This physical practice, combined with spiritual focus, helps prepare your body for restful sleep.

Spirit Renewal Meditation
Spend time in quiet meditation, focusing on the presence of the Holy Spirit within you. Reflect on Romans 8:11, imagining the Spirit filling you with peace and life, refreshing your weary body and mind. As you meditate, let go of any lingering thoughts or anxieties, trusting the Spirit to bring you peace as you sleep.

Scripture Reading for Peace
Before bed, read Romans 8:11 or another comforting scripture. Reflect on how the Holy Spirit, dwelling in you, can provide rest even when you feel restless. Invite the Holy Spirit to be with you as you sleep, bringing renewal and comfort to your body and soul.

Conclusion
Recognizing that God's Spirit dwells within us offers a profound sense of peace and security, especially when we face restless nights or stressful days. Through the Holy Spirit, we are not only empowered for life, but also refreshed and renewed in times of weariness. By embracing the truth that His Spirit lives in you, you can find rest, peace, and clarity, trusting that God will revive and strengthen you each day and night.

Day 13
THE POWER THAT OPERATES WITHIN YOU

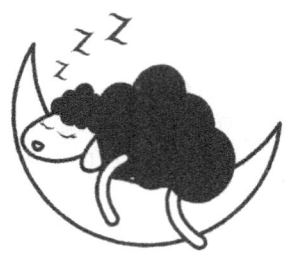

Ephesians 3:20 (KJV):
*"Now unto him that is able to do exceeding abundantly above all
that we ask or think, according to the power that worketh in us."*

The Limitless Power Within You
Imagine you woke up and knew you had a power that you didn't know you had. . .one that is so profound, so immense, beyond anything you could ever ask, or hope for, or even start to think about. It's power that doesn't stand around, but it is living inside you and constantly active in the background and creating amazing things in your life and in the world.

This is no overstatement, and it is also not a fiction. It's who you are in Christ. What works in you is no less than God's own power. Ephesians 3:20 is not just a beautiful scripture to recite on a hushed Sunday morning; it is an explosive declaration of what's possible inside of you. A force strong enough to change your life, to fuel your purpose, and carry you through any situation in the world.

The Power to Overcome
This is the sort of power that enables the impossible. You've got a magical armor and a supernatural power that is not bound by the limits of what you can do or know, when life seems to be going awry, or when the mountain is overwhelming you.

It's not in your strength, your resources, your life experience that this power within you lies. And it's God's power, and there is no boundary to God's power. The same God that made the world is the same God who is inspiring you to get over adversity, face adversity, and accomplish the impossible.

Do you have the experience where you had to take on something and you were like, "this isn't for me." Well, guess what? You do. And not because of anything that happens to you,

Unlock Deep Sleep Secrets

but because of the power that works within you. You'll feel it, and you'll carry it with you when you get frazzled. It will lift you up when you are exhausted. It'll lift you up when you can't get up by yourself.

Much More Than You Can Ask For

What is so lovely about God's grace working in you is that it isn't only for survival, but for success. God's ability to do a thousandfold more than we can think and ask of Him is enumerated in Ephesians 3:20. Take that in for a second.

What are you imagining right now? What are you hoping to get done, what do you hope for, or what would you like to see happen in your life? Whatever it is, God's grace is able to be more. You may have an idea of what you want to be, and that is all that can happen to you, but God's power in you is infinitely bigger than any ideas you might have.

As long as you believe in this strength, you can see higher, achieve bigger, and be bigger. *The might of God in you has no bounds.* It doesn't only satisfy; it outperforms. It's the ability to be something you never imagined.

How This Power Operates

You might ask: What does this power do? What is it doing in my life? What is the solution?

The solution exists through trust and surrender. This force working in you turns on when you let God's power act on you. It's not all about pushing and pulling. It's about being open to the Holy Spirit in you and letting God move through you. Here's how you can get started using that power:

- *Say it's inside of you already.* You don't need to look. Once you became a Christian, you also became a member of the Holy Spirit—the same Spirit that raised Jesus from the dead is now living inside you. This is like you are having access to infinite power, right now.

- *Rely on God's power alone.* And if you're in a rut, know that God can do so much more. Your issues are not big enough for Him. He is stronger than you imagined, to go where you never dreamed.

- *Speak and act in faith.* You can see God at work in your life only by believing. Instill life into the situation, speak the word of God, and walk in faith believing that God will work in you and through you.

- *Surrender to His will.* The power of you unleashed when you place your will into God's. And if you relinquish control, you free up the place for His grace to lead.

31 Days to Overcoming Insomnia

The Power That Fuels Your Purpose
It is not just power for individuality; it is power for mission. God has a purpose for you, and you are the engine that gets you there: The more empowered you are with the Spirit of God, the more prepared you will be to fulfill the calling in your life, to have a difference, to have a legacy.

Every action you take, every choice you make, God is in control within you and working in you to empower and instruct you to do His will. No matter if you're going after your goal, or in a season of struggle, God's will can and will move you forward in the right direction.

Discover the Strength Within You
If you are about to fall asleep this evening, keep this in mind: the force working in you is not a dream; it is now. And you are, right now, infused with infinite power. It is the power of God inside of you that is at work for you.

So as you fall asleep, be at peace in this power. I hope that when you awaken you will experience a day that is powered by God's power, direction, and meaning. You are not alone. The power of God is working in you–performing wonders, breaking down barriers, and making His plans happen in your life.

Remember, as you get out of bed: you are a creature of incomprehensible strength and nothing is impossible for God.

Bask in His strength today and awake to the infinite potential that is waiting for you.

Prayer for the Journey
Dear God, I come to you tonight in admiration of your limitless power and constant love. Ephesians chapter 3 verse 20 is a declaration of your unlimited ability to surpass my expectations and request. As I come to you in prayer tonight, surpass my expectations and go beyond my request and declarations. Soul healer, look into my heart, and see that I have laid before you every concern, every unspoken worry and every restless thought because I know that you are more than able to handle them.

I believe that the same Spirit who raised Christ from the dead is also working on me and restoring my thoughts, body, and soul. Strengthen my heart and mind so that I may fall into deep meditative sleep.

Lord, I acknowledge that Your power is not limited by my understanding or circumstances. You are able to do immeasurably more than I can imagine, and I know that Your power is more than sufficient to re-establish and recharge me as I sleep. I declare that Your strength and peace are at work within me, bringing sound sleep and a refreshed spirit.

Unlock Deep Sleep Secrets

I decree and declare:

Your power is working in me to give me sweet sleep, calm and rejuvenation.
I will have sound sleep, for Jesus is greater than any worry and distress.
I declare I will awake revived, restored and energized by the force within me.
the Lord is doing more than I can think or say, and giving me complete sleep.

I Praise You God, for Your power, which is beyond measure, in me. I'm confident that you can and will give me deep sleep, because you are at work, repairing my body, mind, and spirit. In Jesus' name. Amen.

31 Days to Overcoming Insomnia

JOURNAL
"Sound Sleep is Important"

Morning Journal Guided Reflections

Reflect on a time when you felt God's power working in your life, even in small ways. How did that experience exceed your expectations?

_____
_____
_____
_____
_____

What areas of your life or what restlessness would you like to surrender to God's power?

_____
_____
_____
_____
_____

Write a prayer inviting God to continue working in your life, bringing peace and rest through His unlimited power.

_____
_____
_____
_____
_____

Morning Mindful Rest Practices for Embracing God's Power

Morning Power Prayer
Begin your day with a short prayer, asking God to fill you with His power for the day ahead. As you pray, focus on Ephesians 3:20, remembering that God's power within you is far greater than any challenges you might face.

Scripture Meditation
Read Ephesians 3:20 each morning and spend time meditating on the words "immeasurably more." As you meditate, ask God to reveal to you what "more" He

wants to do in your life—especially in the areas where you feel weak, tired, or overwhelmed.

Morning Affirmation Walk
Take a walk outside or in a peaceful space, and as you walk, repeat to yourself: *"God's power operates in me, doing more than I can imagine."* As you walk, visualize God's power giving you strength, clarity, and peace for the day ahead. This can set a positive, empowering tone for the day.

Power Visualization
Take a few moments in the morning to close your eyes and visualize God's power flowing through you. Picture it as a bright light or wave of energy that fills you with peace and vitality. As you visualize this, imagine how this power will help you overcome the challenges of the day.

Gratitude Journal for God's Power
Start your morning with a gratitude exercise, specifically focusing on ways you've experienced God's power in your life, even in subtle ways. Write down moments where you saw His power helping you or where circumstances worked out better than expected. This practice helps you stay mindful of the power that continues to work within you.

Morning Cognitive Renewal Statements

- God's power operates in me today. Through His strength, I can face every challenge, and He will do more than I can imagine.

Start your day with this affirmation to remind yourself that you are filled with God's power. Speak it aloud or silently, and let it guide you through the challenges of the day with confidence and peace.

Evening Mindful Rest Practices for Resting in God's Power

Evening Reflection on God's Power
Before bed, reflect on the moments of your day where you saw God's power at work, whether through answered prayers, unexpected solutions, or simple peace in moments of stress. Journal about these moments, thanking God for working beyond what you could ask or imagine.

Calming Breath Prayer
Practice a calming breath prayer as you prepare for sleep. Inhale deeply and pray, *"God, Your power works in me,"* then exhale slowly and pray, *"I rest in Your strength."* Repeat

this several times, letting it soothe your mind and body as you prepare to rest, trusting in His power to sustain you.

Progressive Muscle Relaxation with Scripture
As you prepare for bed, lie down and practice progressive muscle relaxation.

Begin with your toes and work your way up to your head, tensing each muscle group and then releasing. As you release, silently pray, *"God's power is at work in me."* This relaxation technique, combined with the affirmation, helps to release physical and mental tension, preparing you for restful sleep.

Visualizing God's Power in Sleep
Spend a few quiet moments before bed visualizing God's power enveloping you as you sleep. Picture a peaceful, protective presence over you, filling your heart and mind with peace and rest. Let go of any anxieties or worries, trusting that God's power will continue to work within you, even as you sleep.

Evening Cognitive Renewal Statements
God's power is at work in me, even as I rest. I release my worries, knowing that He will do more than I can ask or imagine.

Repeat this affirmation before bed as a way to let go of any lingering stress or anxiety. Trust that God's power will continue to work in your life as you sleep, restoring and renewing you for the next day.

Final Thoughts
Knowing and tapping into the power that is inside of you can help you transform how you handle sleep, anxiety, and agitation. We can learn from Ephesians 3:20 that God's strength is unimaginable, and it works in us to do more than we can imagine. Whether you are preparing for a new day or getting ready to fall asleep, know that God's strength is always there to teach, refuel, and empower you. Prayer, contemplation, and mindful practice will allow you to experience the rest and serenity that comes from knowing God's power is working inside of you always.

Day 14
IGNITING YOUR INNER SPARK: THE TRANSFORMATIVE POWER OF SELF-CARE

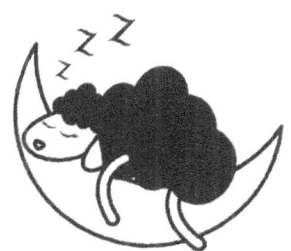

Psalm 127:2 (NIV):
"In vain you rise early and stay up late, toiling for food to eat— for he grants sleep to those he loves."

Life moves fast. We manage jobs, challenges, and don't always stop to be honest with ourselves. Personal self-care is often construed as an expense or an indulgence. But self-care isn't just about pampering yourself from time to time; it's a daily routine that heals your mind, body, and soul. You put yourself at the top of the list so that you shine in your life.

Self-care isn't about avoiding the self; it's about loving yourself deeply and transforming yourself. If we love ourselves, we activate an unrelenting force that makes us more resilient, energized, and aligned with purpose. Be prepared to experience the magic of self-care as we take you through simple but impactful steps that take you off the ground and leave you feeling inspired, positive, and vibrant. God desires for us to practice balance, rest, and trust in His care for us.

Reclaiming Your Time: The Power of Saying "No"
The first step to good self-care is setting limits. We tend to "yes" too often because we have to, or because we don't want to offend anyone. But every time we push ourselves to their limits, we run out of energy and end up burnt out and bitter.

And imagine what your life would be like if you wouldn't take things to heart when you needed to. If you say "no," it's not because you're disrespectful, but because it's good for you. When you reclaim your time and energy, you open the door to the things you care about: sleep, happiness, and what's meaningful to you.

31 Days to Overcoming Insomnia

The Thoughtful Hour: Living in the Moment – Experience It Right Now
We live in a distraction culture, and it is easy to lose yourself in the sound. But when you reconnect with what is here now, that's when you truly start caring about yourself. Mindfulness is the easy but potent practice of paying attention to what you are doing and seeing it all around you.

Mindfulness, whether for a few minutes' deep breathing or drinking a cup of tea, is an effort to disengage yourself from the outside world and engage with yourself. This grounding exercise calms you down, helps you to see things clearly, and lets you deal with the obstacles in your life more comfortably and naturally.

Movement that Makes You Move: Dance & Swing for Your Pleasure!
We usually think of self-care as being physically active, but it's not only going to the gym or walking miles. What is actually self-care? It's moving your body the way YOU feel comfortable with—*w*hether that be dancing in your living room, hiking in the woods, or doing yoga.

Make sure it is a movement you feel like moving, so you feel alive, confident, and connected to your body. It is more than just for the body—regular movement improves your mood, calms your nerves, and awakens your energy. As you move in a way that is happy, you take the tension off of yourself and allow for creativity and understanding to flow.

Nutrition in the Body: *A Fuel for the Soul*
What we put into our mouths either recharges or depletes us. One of the most effective self-care strategies is feeding your body with real foods, rich in nutrients. It's not only about what you eat though, but also how you eat.

Don't rush and try everything in one go without tasting and tasting the flavors. To eat in this way is to engage with your body and its needs and cues. Eat foods that nourish, invigorate, and make you feel good, not only in the present, but also in the future. Your body is your best friend, so treat it with care and attention.

Sleeping With a Purpose: *Power Up Your Batteries*
Sleep, in our hustle-a-day world, has come to be perceived as a privilege or a failure. But the reality is that we need rest to be healthy and balanced. Your body and your brain take time out to refuel, heal, and rehabilitate.

Make rest a priority by adding relaxation to your schedule. Nap, sleep, or do something that gets you back into the groove—whether it's reading a book, taking a bath, or practicing meditation. When you allow yourself to rest, you increase productivity, creativity, and emotional strength.

Unlock Deep Sleep Secrets

Mental Health First: *Finding Inner Peace*
Self-care isn't just about being physically healthy, but about being mentally healthy as well. Mental health is the key to good health. The best mental health regimen keeps you from stress, anxiety, and a loss of your sanity.

You can incorporate practices that encourage mental serenity and focus, like journaling, meditation, or consulting with a therapist. Strike back at negative thoughts and swap them for affirmations of self-love and kindness. Just keep in mind you are not your thoughts; you are the viewer.

Reach out and Connect: *The Power of Relationships to Heal You*
We are social creatures and our connections are critical to our health. Spend your time with people that inspire you, give you support for your ideas, and push you to succeed. Self-care is about being careful about who you invite into your life.

Make room for relationships—with your family, your friends, or in groups of like-minded people. They feed the heart, excite, and offer emotional stability when times are hard. Don't let the therapeutic effect of conversation or laughter be underestimated.

Scriptural Reflection
Psalm 127:2 (NIV): *"In vain you rise early and stay up late, toiling for food to eat—for he grants sleep to those he loves."*

This verse instructs us that we need to put our trust in God's provision and not work ourselves silly. It teaches us that self-care means having boundaries for work and effort, space for sleep, and rest. No amount of late-night work or early morning waking can substitute for the serenity and salvation that come from faith in God. He takes care of us, even in the midst of sleep. When we discipline our lives, we open ourselves to receive the rest that God wills on behalf of His children.

Prayer for the Journey
Dear God, You are the Chief Orchestrator and tonight, I'm grateful for Your care and love. I come before tonight laying down every uneasiness and burden at your feet. Teach me to trust is your provision and how to submit to your authority. Remind me that you are working on my behalf even when I am asleep. Help me to release the need to control and instead embrace the gift of rest you offer.

I know that You have created me with a purpose in mind, and that caring for myself is an important part of fulfilling my God given purpose. Help me to accept the transformative power of self-care and recognize that rest is a vital part of nurturing the inner spark You have given me. I believe that You will guide me to a place of peace, where I can lay down all stress, troubles, and worries, and have a peaceful sleep.

31 Days to Overcoming Insomnia

Lord your word said, **It is vain for you to rise up early, to sit up late, to eat the bread of sorrows;** *therefore, I will not take part in the useless habit of getting up early and staying up late to engage in labor that is accompanied by anxiety and stress, reflecting a life lacking peace. But as you word says,* **for so he giveth his beloved sleep,** *I choose to receive the blessings that you give me, your beloved while I sleep.*

I ask that You help me recognize the importance of myself—physically, mentally, and spiritually. As I nurture myself, may this enable me to live fully for You each day. I decree that my body, mind and spirit are refreshed by the life-giving energy of sleep. I decree that I will sleep well because I know that God will provide comfort for me. I decree God is reviving my spark and preparing me for His will for my life.

I thank You for putting me, your beloved to sleep. I trust that by healing me while I sleep, you are preparing me again for the tasks you've prepared for me. In Jesus' name. Amen.

Unlock Deep Sleep Secrets

JOURNAL
"Sound Sleep is Important"

Morning Journal Guided Reflections

Reflect on your current daily routines. Are there areas where you struggle to practice self-discipline, especially regarding rest and sleep? What changes could you make in your daily schedule to allow for more intentional rest and to trust in God's provision, rather than overworking?

_____
_____
_____
_____
_____
_____
_____
_____
_____
_____
_____
_____

Write a prayer, asking God to help you develop personal self-discipline, trusting Him to provide rest and peace as you follow His wisdom.

_____
_____
_____
_____
_____
_____
_____
_____
_____
_____
_____
_____
_____

31 Days to Overcoming Insomnia

Morning Mindful Rest Practices for Developing Self-Discipline

Morning Routine Planning:
Start your morning by planning your day with intentional time for work, rest, and reflection. List your top three priorities, ensuring that rest and time with God are included. This simple practice encourages self-discipline by setting a clear direction for your day.

Morning Gratitude and Focus Prayer
Before diving into your daily tasks, take time to express gratitude for the rest you received (even if it wasn't perfect) and for the opportunities ahead. Pray for God's guidance to help you maintain balance and self-discipline throughout the day. Thank Him for the gift of sleep and ask for the wisdom to prioritize rest.

Time-Block Scheduling
Implement time blocking in your day to ensure you have moments for work, rest, and personal care. For example, set dedicated time for focused work, a break for physical activity, and an evening wind-down routine. This helps prevent burnout and encourages self-discipline by managing time effectively.

Morning Reflection on Psalm 127:2
Write Psalm 127:2 in your journal or on a note and reflect on how this verse can shape your approach to work and rest today. Allow this Scripture to guide you in practicing self-discipline, ensuring you leave space for the rest that God desires for you.

_____
_____
_____
_____
_____
_____
_____
_____
_____

Mindful Eating Practice
Begin your morning with a nourishing meal, practicing mindfulness in eating. Take time to reflect on how caring for your body with healthy food and habits, rather than rushing through meals, is a form of self-discipline that honors the temple of the Holy Spirit within you.

Unlock Deep Sleep Secrets

Morning Cognitive Renewal Statements

- Today, I will trust in God's provision and practice self-discipline. I will work with intention and rest in His peace.

Start your morning with this affirmation, reminding yourself to approach the day with balanced effort and trust in God's care. By speaking this affirmation, you set the tone for a disciplined, yet peaceful day.

Evening Mindful Rest Practices for Self-Discipline in Rest

Evening Reflection on Work and Rest Balance
Before bed, spend a few moments reflecting on your day. Did you maintain a healthy balance between work and rest? Did you overwork, or were you able to trust God by letting go and winding down?

_____
_____
_____
_____
_____
_____

Journal about what went well and what could be improved tomorrow.

_____
_____
_____
_____
_____
_____

Pre-Bedtime Digital Detox
Practice self-discipline by setting a boundary with technology before bed. Turn off screens at least 30 minutes before sleeping to avoid overstimulation and to allow your mind to settle. Use this time for prayer, reading scripture, or gentle relaxation.

Evening Stretch and Breathe
Create an evening wind-down routine that includes gentle stretching and deep breathing exercises. As you stretch, thank God for the gift of rest and for His provision, even while you sleep. This mindful practice encourages self-discipline by establishing a healthy routine before bed.

31 Days to Overcoming Insomnia

Evening Scripture Reading and Reflection
Read Psalm 127:2 or another calming verse before bed. Reflect on how God's gift of sleep is an act of love and provision for you. Use this time to center your thoughts on God, trusting that He will provide for your needs even as you rest.

Journaling for Self-Discipline
At the end of the day, journal about how well you practiced self-discipline. Did you take time to rest? Did you let go of unnecessary tasks? Write about any areas where you need more discipline and ask God to help you make healthier choices tomorrow.

_____
_____
_____
_____
_____

Evening Cognitive Renewal Statements

- I release my day to God, trusting that He grants me rest. I choose to practice self-discipline by making room for His peace and sleep.

Repeat this affirmation before bed to let go of any lingering work-related thoughts or anxieties. It reinforces the importance of creating space for rest, trusting that God's love and provision continue as you sleep.

Final Thoughts
Practicing personal self-discipline, especially around rest and sleep, is an essential aspect of living a balanced and peaceful life. Psalm 127:2 reminds us that striving without rest is in vain because God is the ultimate provider. By developing habits of discipline, such as managing your time effectively and creating routines for both work and rest, you create space for the rest that God grants to those He loves. Trusting in His provision, you can experience true peace and renewal, allowing both your body and spirit to be restored.

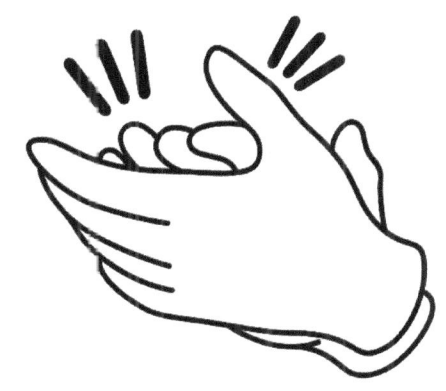

**WAY TO GO!!!
YOU MADE IT THROUGH
14 DAYS OF SLEEP REJUVENATION!**

Day 15
KEEP PUSHING:
THE RELENTLESS POWER OF PERSEVERANCE

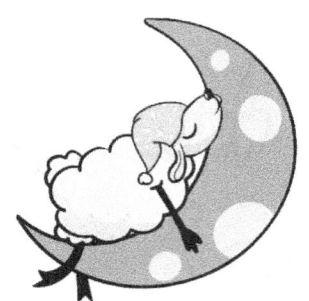

Isaiah 43:2 (NIV):
*"When you pass through the waters, I will be with you;
and when you pass through the rivers, they will not sweep over you."*

There are times in life when it's all or nothing. When the odds seem too much, when obstacles put you at an advantage that you don't know how to continue. These are the moments when it all really becomes magic, when you unleash the power of hard work, break through your own self-imposed limits and prove you're stronger than you thought possible.

As we meditate on the unending strength of endurance, let's look to Isaiah 43:2, which provides an abundance of encouragement: *"When you pass through the waters, I will be with you; and when you pass through the rivers, they will not overtake you. When you go through the fire, you will not burn; the fire will not burn you."* These words assure us that we are never truly alone, no matter how difficult things seem to be. Even when we are at our craziest, we are encouraged and encouraged to keep going.

And that verse isn't only a prayer for survival; it's a declaration of strength, for endurance, for unflinching hope. It tells us that however high the waters rise, however fierce the flames burn, **we are unstoppable with God by our side.** Let's talk about what it means to continue fighting when the odds are against us and how we can draw on this God-given strength that keeps us going through all of our struggles.

The Seas: Overcoming All Obstacles
It's like being on the sea's edge, the ocean battering your shore. The sea is dark and slippery, tugging at your feet, trying to sweep you away. This is what many of us experience when

Unlock Deep Sleep Secrets

confronted with seemingly impossible life challenges. Whether that's stress, loss, heartbreak, or money, it's as though the whole world is pulling down on us and we barely survive.

The exciting part, though, is that God has already avowed that you will not be swept up! The first half of Isaiah 43:2 reads *"When you pass through the waters, I will be with you."* Notice the important phrase: *"When you pass through."* It's not as if you pass through. Not that we'll have problems, but they will. But God's Word is unfailing: He will stand by you, and you will emerge from it more empowered than ever.

Keep pushing through the waters. Maybe you're floating in the water, but God is holding you, supporting you, and steering you through the most challenging storms. Don't stop swimming. Don't stop fighting. With God on your side, there is no wave that you cannot surmount. Each thing that comes against you is your chance to experience His power, to overcome, and to triumph.

The Rivers: Unbending Strength in the River of Life

Now imagine that you are in the middle of a flowing stream. The current is fast, the water swift, and every movement tries to push you down. The river never stops and yet, no matter how hard you push, it just pushes you back. Life's troubles are not, sometimes, individual, intermittent ones; they are unceasing, unflinching, persistent: sucking us under, tumbling over and twirling away.

But God says, *"The rivers will not overwhelm you."* Rivers might be coming, but they will not flood you. You might feel the rush, but God's power is bigger in you. The river of life may want to drown you, but it cannot.

Continue slogging through your own life's streams. You might be tired, but every single step, however small, is a victory. The water may be deep, but you are brighter, and God is directing your every step. With Him at your side, the river may push you down, but it can never drown you. Your power is in Him, and He will get you through to the other side.

The Burn: Coming Through Redeemed and Undamaged

Fire is the thing that truly pushes our boundaries. Fire symbolizes the calamities that arise—those which seemingly devour everything that passes and threaten to shatter us from within. From personal hurt, crushing losses, or seemingly impossible challenges, the heat can become unbearable. The fires chase us and it's like the fire will devour us all.

But here's the heartening thing about Isaiah 43:2: *"You will not be burned; the fire will not burn you alive."* You might feel like you're entering a furnace, but you won't burn. You are not just being spared by the fire; you are thriving under it, and God's protection is a wall around you.

31 Days to Overcoming Insomnia

Remember the biblical tale of Shadrach, Meshach, and Abednego being thrown into a burning furnace for not worshipping a devil. When they were tossed into the fire, it was not death, but divine redemption. Not only were they safe, but the king even saw a fourth man walking alongside them in the fire, and it was God Himself. Their fire did not devour them; it revealed to the world just how alive and present God is amid our suffering.

Keep walking in the fire, for in the fire your faith is sharpened, your nature created, and your confidence in God becomes unbreakable. Fire may surround you, but they can't reach you. You'll exit the flames not as a victim, but as a winner—cleaned, restored, and renewed by the presence of God.

The Strength of Denial: God's Word Is Inviolable

Isaiah 43:2 speaks universally of divine perseverance. Waters, streams, and fires exist, and we will see them. But even in each of these struggles, God's Word is evident: we are not going to be defeated.

The wonderful thing about this promise is that it is not only about surviving—it is about growing from it. It's about knowing that God's presence is not just a passive consolation, but a powerful presence that lives within us, inspires us, and leaves us unconquerable. Pushing is not just staying alive, but becoming who God has designed us to be, stronger, braver, more resilient every time.

Keep pushing forward. Life doesn't drown you. Be careful of the rivers. Don't burn yourself out by the fire. If God is with you, you'll be okay. Each hurdle is preparation for another, and every movement is a victory march.

Prayer for the Journey

Dear God, I come before You tonight, tired but hopeful, believing that You keep me alive despite all the trials and hardships I encounter. As I rest, I trust Your word in Isaiah 43:2, that whatever waters I tread, no matter what fires I suffer, you are with me.

Please give me the courage to keep going, even when the day's burden is overwhelming. Turn off my thoughts of fear and tell me I'm not alone in this fight for good rest and sweet sleep. It is you who separates the seas before me and protects me from the flames that are ready to destroy me. Therefore, I Put the rattling of my mind to rest in Jesus' name. You are my God who opens seas and make a way before me. You are my God who and saves me from the fires which come to consume me.

Lord, as this day comes to a close, take my effort and substitute it with faith, my fatigue with serenity, and my skepticism with absolute certainty. Soothe my heart with the promise that You're with me, that You are always there, and every breathe I take in sleep is a breath of refreshment from you.

Unlock Deep Sleep Secrets

Tonight, I decree that I am armed with the Lord through every moment of this night. Therefore, as I Walk through waters and fiery trials I will not drown or perish. God is in my midst, and He is my shield.

Isaiah chapter 43 verse 2 reminds me that no matter how overwhelming life may feel, whether through the stresses of daily life, challenges in relationships, or moments of fear, God is always with me, ensuring that I am never alone

Nothing will hinder my journey to attain refreshing sleep, for I am held by the unfailing hand of Jesus. My Heart and mind are at ease, and when I lay down, I will get regenerative rest for the next day.

I decree my bedtime will be restful tonight. I owe everything to God and rise with new optimism and relentless determination. In Jesus' name, I pray. Amen.

31 Days to Overcoming Insomnia

JOURNAL
"Sound Sleep is Important"

Morning Cognitive Renewal Statements

Affirmation of God's Promise

What promise of God do I need to remember today? (e.g., "When you pass through the waters, I will be with you.")
___
___
___

How can I actively trust God with this promise today?
___
___
___

Morning Journal Guided Reflections

Embrace God's Presence
What challenge or opportunity am I facing today that I need God's help with?
___
___
___

How can I invite God's presence into this situation, knowing He is with me through every trial?
___
___
___

Strength for the Day Ahead
What do I need strength for today? How can I rely on God's strength to keep me going through the day's struggles?
___
___
___

Unlock Deep Sleep Secrets

Set Your Intentions
What is one thing I can do today to keep pushing forward, even when the going gets tough?

_____
_____
_____

How will I remind myself to keep going, even in moments of doubt or difficulty?

_____
_____
_____

Morning Prayer and Imagination: Morning Mindful Rest Practice (5-10 Minutes)

Deep Breathing and Prayer
- Just sit quietly and breathe slowly for four seconds, hold four, and let go for four. Try this for a few minutes to quiet your mind and your heart.
- Then, say a prayer to draw God into your life: *"God, thank you for being with me in this moment. Give me faith today to believe in Your promises and empower me to conquer what I am facing. And I know I can beat it, no matter how strong it might be, with You."*

Visualization of Strength
Close your eyes and imagine yourself facing a challenge today, but this time imagine yourself with God by your side. Think of Him holding your hand, encouraging you through each step, leading you when things feel like crap.

Say this to yourself during the vision: *"God is with me, I can keep walking."*

Morning Cognitive Renewal Statements
As you close your morning journal, reaffirm your confidence in God's Word:

- I will keep on pushing today because God has my back when I have any challenge.
- I believe that the power of God is my power, and no test shall shake me.
- The rivers, the fires and the waters will not overwhelm me; I will triumph with God.
- I'm not weak, I'm not weakened, and I am not broken, because God is with me today.

31 Days to Overcoming Insomnia

Evening Journal Guided Reflections

Reflect on the Day
What waters, rivers, or fires did I face today? How was I led by God through those struggles? What moments today made me feel overwhelmed, and how did I endure it with God's help?

_____
_____
_____
_____
_____

How can I be thankful today, even in the midst of pain?

_____
_____
_____
_____
_____
_____

How did God be so faithful today, and how did He move me out of my problems?

_____
_____
_____
_____
_____
_____

Acknowledge Your Progress

How did I grow today?

_____
_____
_____
_____
_____

So, what small victories have I won and how do I recognize my growth towards overcoming obstacles?

_____
_____
_____
_____
_____

Unlock Deep Sleep Secrets

What talents have I discovered in myself today that I had not considered?
_____
_____
_____
_____

Prepare for Tomorrow

So, what's on my agenda tomorrow?
_____
_____
_____
_____
_____

How can I prepare myself for them with faith and power?
_____
_____
_____
_____
_____

How will I be able to place God's faith in tomorrow's trials and expect Him to support me?
_____
_____
_____
_____
_____

Evening Mindful Rest Practice:
Guided Relaxation and Visualization to Achieve Sleep Calm (5-10 Minutes)

Guided Relaxation
You lay down in a peaceful room. You should breathe long, slowly, uninhibited, and let go of the tension in your body as you breathe in and out. Take a breath and let go of the worries or stresses in your head. Imagine God surrounding you, calming you, pacifying you.

31 Days to Overcoming Insomnia

Visualization of God's Protection
Imagine yourself again standing in the rivers or fires of your day, but this time with God's shield surrounding you. You are never hurt by Him and the things you endured today could never hurt you.

Recite this silently: *I know that God is protecting me and I'm safe in His hands.*

Evening Cognitive Renewal Statements

Let these affirmations encapsulate your mind and soul at the end of your nighttime meditation:
- God is on my side and I am in His care. I can rest assured He will not hurt me.
- I will go to sleep knowing God is with me and that I am never alone in my battle.
- It is God's turn tomorrow, and I am relying on Him to take care of whatever comes my way.
- I'm powerful, resilient and peaceful, knowing God's love and power are always there.

Day 16
MY MOUTH WILL SPEAK LIFE

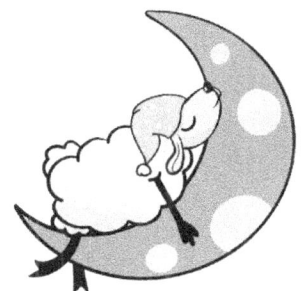

Proverbs 18:21 (NIV):
*"Life and death are in the power of the tongue,
and those who love it will eat its fruit."*

As we've all heard, "Sticks and stones may break my bones, but words will never hurt me." This is a good saying, but it could not be any truer. Words make our world, our feelings, and even our sleep. We are told in Proverbs 18:21 that "The tongue is life and death, and those who love it will eat its fruit." Our words aren't just sounds; they are seeds, which can nourish or harm, heal or kill, soothe or stir.

When it comes to sleep, what we say to ourselves, to others, and to our world is how much we can determine whether we sleep soundly or unsoundly. With the words life–affirmations, thoughts, conscious words–we can literally modify our state of mind and emotions so as to allow sleep that is not only restful but deeply restorative.

Words Can Make a Difference for A Peaceful Night's Sleep

When we use words of life, we're creating a space for peace. We are brains and bodies–and words are the link. Talking in the affirmative increases neurotransmitters such as serotonin and oxytocin, which ease stress and anxiety, so that we feel more at peace. But when we talk about negative things, like worry or fear–and we tend to say these things in the middle of the night–our brain does keep a ticking clock and we can't sit still.

In the sleep world, it stands to reason: what you tell yourself at night is either the thing that settles your brain for a deep sleep, or it is the thing that sends you twitching and screaming in bed.

31 Days to Overcoming Insomnia

The function of Self-Talk During Sleep
Have you ever been trying to go to sleep after a long day of stress or anxiety? Or maybe you think all about it and replay the day, the conversation, the anxiety. That is usually caused by negative thoughts or unacknowledged feelings. What we tell ourselves when we lie down at night is important because either peace or conflict are sparked by it.

If your mind chatters "I'll never get enough sleep," or "I can't sleep because my brain is too busy," you are feeding the very problem you're trying to prevent. But if you prefer to sleep with the words of life, then your body and mind will start to unwind. Begin meditating on statements like:

- I am calm, my body is relaxed, and I am ready for a good night's sleep.
- Being asleep is my way, and I deserve to sleep.

This type of self-talk will all help set the stage for sleep to be the inevitable outcome.

How Speaking Life Promotes Restful Sleep
The language we speak serves as a map of the mind and heart that takes us through the day, and even more so, the night. Here are some examples of how you can breathe life into your sleep habit to directly enhance the quality of your sleep:

Calming the Mind
Things get negative, worries start running around our heads when there is not much going on outside of our minds, we cannot be calm. But affirmation and thanksgiving can reorient you. When you intentionally say 'yes', you are moving your mind to harmony and relaxation and telling your body to chill out. Do not let fear occupy you, but instead, say phrases of calm:

- I am not in danger and I am not troubled.
- I give up today and let rest replenish me.
- My body is quiet, and my mind is quiet.
- Sleep is beautiful, organic stuff.

Releasing Tension
As we resound encouragement and affirmation, we also call up a physical release of tension in our bodies. Suppose you say to yourself, *"I am worthy of rest"*, with a slow exhalation. Your joints will relax, your heart rate will slow and your body will go easy. Sayings such as "I give up all stress and allow peace" invite the body to let go of physical stress that may interfere with sleep.

Unlock Deep Sleep Secrets

Creating a Positive Sleep Environment
Your bedroom is where the energy is important to you. What is your TV room about? Are you taking it as a home or a place to truly unwind, or do you take it as a frustration saying, "I can't sleep in here?" If you talk into your room, you give it life. Try saying:

- I have a bedroom where I can relax and be at peace.
- My body and my mind can sleep here.
- I thank God for my bed, and I let myself sleep.

When you set your space as a place where you'll be calm and happy, your mind will be drawn to that meaning, so you can relax and go to sleep.

Prayer for the Journey
Dear God, I thank You for the wisdom of Proverbs 18:21, which reminds me of the power of my words. Tonight, I choose to speak life and align my words with Your promises. I reject fear, anxiety, and negative thoughts, and I declare that Your peace and rest are mine.

As I lay down to sleep tonight, I thank You for what my words can and can't do. My tongue is an instrument of life and death, I am reminded of Your Word in Proverbs 18:21 "Life and death are in the power of the tongue, and those who love it will eat its fruit". This scripture affirms that there is power in my words. Therefore, I am making a deliberate decision this evening to promote sweet sleep, I am speaking life over myself, my present, and my future.

Lord, I decree my words are going to be according to Your truth. I replace all the bad thoughts and swap them for life-giving words of hope, peace, and faith. Since what I say can affect my mental and emotional state and prevent me from getting a good night's sleep, I guard my tongue even when I am unsure so that I can sow seeds of abundance and not discouragement.

At this moment, I choose to silence the inner voice of fear, panic, anxiety, unforgiveness, worry, defeat, and anything that weighs me down and focus on things that are pure and of a good report.

- *I decree that my words will be life-changing.*
- *I decree that when I lay my head down to sleep it will be sweet.*
- *I decree that because Jesus is my Jehovah Rapha I'm healed emotionally and physically of any pain and will not be awaken by any discomfort and worry.*
- *I decree God gives me rest because he loves me*

31 Days to Overcoming Insomnia

- *I decree the Lord leads me beside still waters and restores my soul.*
- *I decree I lay down in peace and safety for the Lords watches over my soul.*
- *I decree I cast all my anxieties on God for he cares for me.*
- *I decree the Lord is my keeper. He watches over me while I sleep.*
- *I decree God gives me peace that surpasses all understanding and he guards my heart and mind to sweet sleep tonight.*

Thank you for the joy that comes with articulating life and knowing that, in so doing, I'm creating a positive attitude and environment for healing to flow while I rest. Tonight, I will sleep peacefully, and wake up refreshed, ready to speak life again. In Jesus' name, I pray. Amen.

Unlock Deep Sleep Secrets

JOURNAL
"Sound Sleep is Important"

Morning Cognitive Renewal Statements

- I declare that my words today will speak life, hope, and peace. I trust in God's strength and His peace that surpasses understanding. In quietness, I find my rest.
- My mouth will speak life, and I will see the fruit of my faith in every area of my life. Mountains of doubt, stress, and fear are removed as I declare God's promises.

Morning Journal Guided Reflections

What words do I want to speak over my life today? Write a life-giving affirmation to set the tone for the day.

_____
_____
_____
_____

What areas of my life I need God's peace and strength?

_____
_____
_____
_____

How can I align my words with God's promises for those areas?

_____
_____
_____
_____

Morning Mindful Rest Practice

Breathing and Speaking Life
Sit quietly for 5 minutes, focusing on your breath. Inhale deeply through your nose, hold for a few seconds, and then exhale slowly through your mouth. As you exhale, speak softly, *"I breathe in peace, and I breathe out stress."* Repeat this, alternating with *"My mouth speaks life."*

31 Days to Overcoming Insomnia

Verbal Gratitude List
After your breathing exercise, verbally list three things you are grateful for.

- I am grateful for _____
- I am thankful for _____
- I appreciate _____

Evening Cognitive Renewal Statements

- Tonight, I release any burdens or negative words I've spoken or heard today. I embrace God's rest, and I declare peace over my mind and body. I trust God to work in every area of my life as I sleep.
- I am free from anxiety. I speak life and peace over my sleep. My rest will be deep and renewing.

Evening Journal Guided Reflections

What words did I speak today that brought life?
_____
_____
_____
_____

How did they impact my mood or interactions with others?
_____
_____
_____
_____

Were there any words I spoke that might have brought harm or negativity?
_____
_____
_____
_____

How can I replace them with words of faith and peace?
_____
_____
_____
_____

Unlock Deep Sleep Secrets

Evening Mindful Rest Practices

- **Quiet Reflection**
Before bed, take a few moments to reflect on your day. Think about the words you've spoken—were they life-giving or fear-filled?

_____
_____
_____

If there were any negative words or thoughts, repent of them and ask God for His peace to replace them. Speak aloud, *"I cancel any negative words I've spoken today, and I declare peace over my mind."*

- **Scripture Meditation**
Repeat Isaiah 30:15 slowly, letting the words sink in: *"In quietness and trust is my strength."* Allow this verse to shape your thoughts before you sleep. Let God's quietness bring rest to your spirit.

Weekly Reflection

Reflect on how your words have impacted your sleep over the week. Were there days where you felt more at peace?

_____
_____
_____
_____

How did speaking life change your outlook and rest?

_____
_____
_____
_____

Day 17
DREAM IT TO EXISTENCE

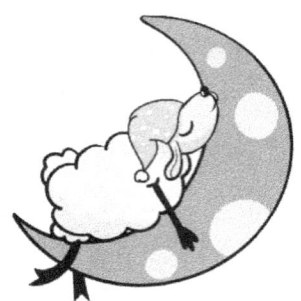

Exodus 33:14 (NIV):
"My presence will go with you, and I will give you rest."

We all dream, don't we? I want to be a better person and have a life that's worthwhile, that's successful, and that's fulfilling. But sometimes, these dreams are just that, dreams that are distant and inaccessible. For a promise that can alter dreams and sleep: "My feet will follow you, and I will put your sleep to rest." Exodus 33:14 is so true.

And this verse isn't a just a promise of peace that God will be there, but to dream big and sleep soundly that God will be here with us. Suppose you are dreaming it to life in the daytime, and sleeping sound, restful sleep in the evening, all because you believe in God's direction and calm. It is the life that God will give to His people who believe. When He goes with us, our imagination brims with life, and we fall asleep like never before.

Dreaming with God's Presence, the Authority of Dreaming with God
Moses had enormous problems when he took the Israelites into the wilderness. But God had promised to be with him and that made all the difference. Moses wasn't stranded alone in the unknown. He had God all around him, his helper, his bulwark, his guide and his calm.

And so too, in dreaming it into being, we are never alone. We're walking with the same God who walked with Moses in the desert. When we dream together with God, we are not just dreaming a future for ourselves; we are creating dreams according to His purpose and trusting that He will guide us to put them into action.

Dreaming with God is surrender and giving Him the time and the place. This collaboration frees us from pressure, from doing all the work, and from the fear of "how" our hopes will be

Unlock Deep Sleep Secrets

realized. And that is where rest is necessary. This rest is not from bodily fatigue, but also from the emotional and psychological strain of stress and endeavor.

The Rest of God: Silent Sleep as a Sight of Hope—Sound Sleep is the Vision of Justice

We think of rest as the time away from doing, but in Scripture, rest is so much more. Then, in Exodus 33:14, God says not only physical rest, but also inner rest—a rest in which we no longer fear and worry, particularly at night, when we should be resting.

Its association with dreaming it to life and peaceful sleep is powerful. As long as we can believe God, then we can rest in His promises, and we can do the same when we fall asleep. Ask yourself: How many times a night are you up, with your mind filled with the nitty-gritty of everything you have to get done or the questions about the future? The counterweight to this anxiety is slumber by God.

When we dream with God, we leave the doubt about the outcome at the door, and trust in the power of His enactment. This faith leads to a sound sleep because our dreams are His and He is in control, and all is good.

Healthy sleep is not merely physical—it is spiritual. When we're peaceful with God, we sleep—and rest nourishes our body, mind, and soul so that we're ready for the next day.

Prayer for the Journey

Dear God, thank you for the promise you made in Exodus chapter 33 and verse 14, reminding me that your presence will go with me and you will give me rest. Thank you for your presence which assures me that you are personally with me, guiding and protecting me on this journey to achieve sweet sleep. Thank you for the promise of your rest, both physical and spiritual. While my body rests from the challenges thrown at me by the enemy, my spirit also rests in your security and care.

Tonight, I release myself from restlessness that comes from trying to carry burdens that God never intended for me to bear alone. I surrender these burdens and embrace the rest that comes from trusting in God's presence.

As I sleep, I rest in the confidence that you are working all things together for my good. Thank you once again for this awesome promise of your guaranteed presence and the peace the passes all understanding. Wow, I can already feel sweet sleep is about to sweep over me.

I decree sweet sleep is my portion, my heart will be relaxed, and I will wake up fresh and full of new strength. You are the God who is the giver of dreams as well as the giver of life. Tonight, I rest my head and heart in Your everlasting arms, because You're well able to finish what You began in me. In Jesus' name, I pray. Amen.

31 Days to Overcoming Insomnia

JOURNAL
"Sound Sleep is Important"

Morning Cognitive Renewal Statements

- Today, I dream with confidence and faith. I trust that God's presence is with me as I take steps toward bringing my dreams into existence.
- I have faith in the unseen, and I know that what I hope for is coming to life. God's presence guides me, and I trust Him to fulfill the dreams He has placed in my heart.

Morning Journal Guided Reflections

What dream am I believing God for today?

_____
_____
_____
_____
_____

How can I invite His presence into the steps I take toward this dream?

_____
_____
_____
_____
_____

What is one small step I can take today to move closer to bringing my dream to existence?

_____
_____
_____
_____
_____

Morning Mindful Rest Practices

- **Faith-Filled Dream Visualization**
  Take a few moments in the morning to close your eyes and imagine your dream as though it has already come to pass.

Unlock Deep Sleep Secrets

Visualize it vividly, seeing yourself living in that dream. As you visualize, say aloud, *"God's presence is with me, and I have faith that this dream will come to existence."* Feel the confidence and peace that comes with trusting in God's plan.

- **Daily Dream Step**

  Write down what your desires/goals are concerning a perfect sleep. Next to it, write one small action you have taken or will take today that will bring you closer to that dream of a perfect sleep.

  Speak an affirmation over this step, such as: *"I trust that this step is a part of God's plan, and I am moving closer to my dream with every action I take."* Keep this affirmation in mind throughout the day.

Goal

_____
_____
_____
_____
_____
_____
_____

Action I Will Take

_____
_____
_____
_____
_____
_____
_____

Evening Cognitive Renewal Statements

- As I rest tonight, I trust that God is working on my dreams even while I sleep. I release my worries and surrender my plans into His hands, knowing that His presence brings me peace.
- I have faith that my dreams are safe with God. I rest in the assurance that He is guiding me, and I will wake up refreshed and ready to take another step toward my vision.

31 Days to Overcoming Insomnia

Evening Journal Guided Reflection

How did I nurture my dream today?

_____
_____
_____
_____
_____
_____

What actions did I take in faith?

_____
_____
_____
_____
_____
_____
_____

What do I need to release to God tonight so I can rest, trusting Him to guide my dreams into existence?

_____
_____
_____
_____
_____
_____
_____

Evening Mindful Rest Practices

- **Release and Dream**
  Before bed, take a few moments to reflect on your dreams and the steps you took today to move closer to them. Pray this prayer: *"Lord, I give my dreams to You. I trust that You are working in the unseen, and I rest in Your presence tonight. Help me to wake up with renewed faith and vision."*

- **Meditate on Hebrews 11:1**
  As you prepare to sleep, repeat Hebrews 11:1 to yourself: *"Faith is confidence in what we hope for and assurance about what we do not see."* Let these words fill you with peace, trusting that your dreams are being brought to life through your faith and God's guidance. Allow this assurance to calm your heart as you fall asleep.

Unlock Deep Sleep Secrets

Weekly Reflection

Reflect on how your faith has grown as you've held onto your dreams this week. How has trusting in God's presence helped you stay focused and hopeful?

_____
_____
_____

What progress have you made toward your vision?

_____
_____
_____
_____

"Dream It to Existence" in Practice

When you dream with faith and align your vision with God's will, you begin to turn your hopes into reality. Trusting that God's presence goes with you allows you to take bold steps during the day and rest peacefully at night, knowing that He is working behind the scenes to bring your dreams to fruition. By focusing on your dreams and trusting in what is unseen, you can find both motivation and peace, helping you achieve restful, restorative sleep.

Day 18
REFRESHING REST

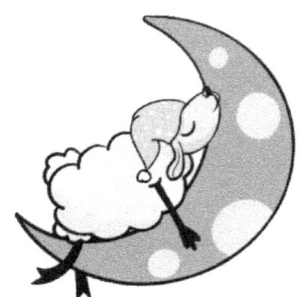

Jeremiah 31:25-26 (NIV):
*"I will refresh the weary and satisfy the faint.
At this I awoke and looked around.
My sleep had been pleasant to me."*

Have you ever woken up feeling tired and groggier than you were when you slept? The day's baggage hangs, you didn't get a rest after all. And if the world is always asking us to do more, you'll start to feel burnt out both mentally and physically. The bustle, the pressure, the unchecked list—you're never quite out of it sometimes. But what if rest is not just sleep? And what if refreshing rest is that rest God Himself promises, a rest that fills you up to the brim, not only in body, but in soul?

The Promise of Refreshing Rest
God's Word doesn't promise a fix, like a few hours of rest; it promises restorative restitution far greater. Cool rest occurs when you let God's love get inside the weary part of your heart. It's the kind of rest that doesn't relax you, but gives you life, and will fill you with God's tranquility and power.

The following verse in Jeremiah then describes the reaction of a person to this spiritual rest: For they went out and were made well: There was no other rest for the gods, and he took him up. "So, I woke up and went about. I'd been sleeping well."

Notice that this isn't just any sleep. It is not staying up all night and getting up tired. This is the type of rest that will make you utterly renewed, as if you have felt a stone lifted off your back. You not only wake up feeling refreshed physically, but spiritually and emotionally too. Your heart is still, and your head is clear.

Unlock Deep Sleep Secrets

Why We Need Refreshing Rest

Why then do we need such rest? We're so tapped-out and worn-out from the demands of life. Physical rest is vital, but so is emotional and spiritual rest. We're not always so fatigued because we don't sleep. At times, it's because of a burden of daily routines, worry, the emotional costs of love, the psychological burden of juggling all this. We are in a world that is all about the hustle and being busy, but when we live like that, we are cut off from our real source of power.

God understands this. He is in the know of how tired you are. And He knows that there is no physical sleep that can get you back to your best without your soul also sleeping. And that is why He has promised to wake up the tired and calm the weak. ... Refreshing sleep is not sleep, but God's divine renewal, so every inch of you is calm, hopeful, and strong.

How to Receive Refreshing Rest

If God promised rest to the tired, how can we get such rest in return? It requires intentionality and trust. How to expose yourself to God's promise of re-nourishing rest here are some ways to make this happen:

Rest in God's Presence

But the only rest comes from believing in God. We sleep like we're asleep —but God's sleeping is never idle. It's just dropping everything and asking God to supply, keep, and reclaim you. To sleep in God is to recognize that He's in charge and that you don't rest on your situation but on His goodness.

Scripture to reflect on: *"Come to me, all you who labour and are heavy-laden, and I will lay your feet down"* (Matthew 11:28).

Surrender Your Burdens

The trick to a newfound rest is letting go. Attempting to bear life's burden alone exhausts us. But when we entrust it to God, we give Him the burden. Such surrender leaves time for His peace to invade our hearts and minds.
Everyday take a few minutes to slow down, close your eyes, and put your anxieties in God's hands. Acknowledge you can't have it all, but He's got you and He's going to get you through it.

Scripture to reflect on: *"All your worries put on him because he loves you."* (1 Peter 5:7).

Make Time for Spiritual Rejuvenation

You sleep, but spiritual resting is the secret of revivifying rest. Spend time in your day praying, reading Scripture, or sitting quietly. In those times, you let God re-energize you. And you may not always be relieved right away, but by seeking God and praying a prayer that God's peace will come over you.

31 Days to Overcoming Insomnia

Scripture to reflect on: *"The Lord strengthens his people; the Lord gives his people rest."* (Psalm 29:11).

Embrace God's Promise
In Jeremiah 31:25-26, we are promised that God will rest the dry and the lame. Believe in that promise! It's so tempting to think that we need to do a lot of work to sleep, or that we need to work ourselves up, or that we must repair ourselves before we can ever recharge. But God's rest is for free. Embrace it! Make sure that when you go to Him, He gives you rest that feeds all your souls.

The Fruit of Refreshing Rest
When we have refreshing rest, we don't just feel better for a while; we are transformed. We sleep with God because God is our power to tackle life in peace and clarity. It recharges us to love better, serve better, and live with purpose. Refreshing rest isn't a moment off; it is the seed of a life lived in God's peace and power.

Your Invitation to Divine Rest
God wants you to live in a state of refreshing sleep. And He promises you today, now. When you're physically worn down, mentally worn down, or spiritually worn down, you get God's rest. He will renew you, give you the rest of your heart, and bring you rest. It's not a rest that disappears —it is a rest that comes back, restores, and renews. And when you wake up, just as the prophet, from this divine sleep, you will look around and see that your soul is regenerated, your spirit renewed, and your sleep has been a good one, because you rest with God. Go and sleep in His word and have the refreshing sleep God wishes you to have. He is ready to save you—body, soul, and spirit.

Prayer for the Journey
Dear God, it's me again coming to You this evening before laying down to sleep. Thank you for Your promise to refresh me when I am tired and strengthen me when I am weak. Paps, just like You gave Jeremiah sweet sleep after revealing Your plans of restoration, I ask that You grant me the same sweet sleep and peace tonight.

Let Your water of the promises of Your word wash over me like a river, soothing all my thoughts and heart. Bring stillness into the depths of my soul so I may rest as refreshingly as possible. I lay the day's burden in Your hands and allow Your Spirit to cleanse me as I fall asleep.

May tonight be one of rest that only You can bring – rest that lifts my soul, restores my intellect, and heals my body. I believe that You are in me while I sleep, cleaning up and shutting down wasteful thoughts entertained throughout the day. I lay down in Your arms knowing I'll wake with new strength and reassurance.

Unlock Deep Sleep Secrets

I decree that tiredness cannot overpower me, for I lie in the arms of the One who cleanses and rehydrates. I will wake up every day reenergized and filled with gratitude.

I surrender my exhaustion to You, knowing that true rest comes from You alone. Thank you for being my refuge, my strength, and my peace. As I close my eyes, I decree, I receive the gift of sweet and peaceful sleep knowing that you are watching over me. In Jesus' name, I pray. Amen.

31 Days to Overcoming Insomnia

JOURNAL
"Sound Sleep is Important"

Morning Cognitive Renewal Statements

- Today, I move forward with a spirit that has been refreshed by God's presence. I trust that He will give me the strength and peace I need to face the day.
- I am fully rested, both in body and spirit. God has refreshed me, and I am ready to embrace today with renewed energy and faith.

Morning Journal Guided Reflections

What am I grateful for this morning that brings me a sense of refreshment and renewal?

_____
_____
_____

How can I allow God's presence to guide me today and continue to refresh my spirit?

_____
_____
_____

Morning Mindful Rest Practices

Breathing in Refreshment
Begin your day with a simple breathing exercise. As you inhale, imagine that you are breathing in God's refreshment and strength. As you exhale, release any lingering tension or worry. Say to yourself, *"God refreshes my soul, and I breathe in His peace."*

Gratitude and Renewal
Write down three things you are grateful for today that make you feel renewed. These can be simple blessings like a peaceful night's sleep, the sound of birds outside, or the warmth of the morning sun. As you reflect on these blessings, thank God for refreshing your spirit and carry that sense of renewal with you throughout the day

- I am grateful or _____
- I am thankful for _____
- I appreciate _____

Unlock Deep Sleep Secrets

Evening Cognitive Renewal Statements

- As I prepare for sleep, I trust that God will refresh my soul and give me rest. I release all my worries to Him and embrace the peace that comes with His presence.
- I rest in God's care, knowing that He will refresh my spirit tonight. My sleep will be pleasant, and I will wake up renewed and strengthened.

Evening Journal Guided Reflections

In what ways did I feel refreshed today by God's presence? How did He renew my strength?

_____
_____
_____
_____

What concerns or burdens do I need to release to God tonight so I can experience true, refreshing rest?

_____
_____
_____
_____

Evening Mindful Rest Practices

Release and Rest
Before bed, take a moment to reflect on anything that may be weighing on your mind or heart. Write down these concerns in your journal, then say a short prayer: *"Lord, I release these worries into Your hands. I trust that You will refresh my soul as I sleep, and I will wake up renewed and rested."* Let go of the burdens as you go to sleep.

Gratitude Meditation
Before you drift off to sleep, think about something from the day that made you feel peaceful or renewed. Focus on that feeling of gratitude and let it wash over you. Say quietly to yourself, *"I am thankful for the refreshing rest God will provide tonight."* Allow that peace to guide you into restful sleep.

Day 19
SURRENDER AND REST

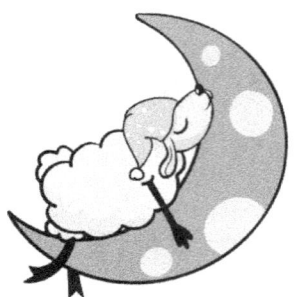

Psalm 62:1 (NIV):
"Truly my soul finds rest in God; my salvation comes from him."

Understanding the Rest of Surrender

Biblical rest isn't sitting back, but submitting ourselves to God's sufficient grace and letting Him carry us. Our psalmist declares in 62:1: "My soul rests in God." That rest is where our anxieties, anxieties, and power go. Surrender is hard to say, but it is the path to an unknowable peace.

Give up: giving up on the power we can't have and letting God do the driving. It's knowing that no matter how hard we try, God alone can keep us at peace and deliver us from evil. Not lying down means being idle. It is resting on God to see that He will take care of us, give us strength, and make us new again when we're exhausted.

And when we give up, God is doing the heavy lifting. It gives us the possibility of a silence that animates instead of sucks.

The Refreshing Force of Rest in God

The real rest is not a nap or vacation; it is in God. It's the kind of rest that renews the spirit — our most tired parts. We're all physically worn out, but the soul weariness is what renders us totally worn. Rest in God is the answer.

When we hand over our troubles to God, that doesn't mean the troubles disappear. But it does end up being the world that we no longer take on. So, we can surrender, so that we can sleep easy and know God will take care of what we cannot. It's knowing God is working, even in the midst of the frenzies. When we decide to put our hearts in the hands of God, He

Unlock Deep Sleep Secrets

restores us, He heals us and leaves us peaceful. And it's not just an hour's rest, but a soul-centered peace that lasts through the day, through the difficulties, and into the night.

Prayer for the Journey

Dear God, As I prepare to sleep this evening, quiet my heart and soothe my mind. Let Your peace surrounds me like a shield, protecting me from anxious thoughts that cause restless nights. Your word in Psalms 61:1 reminds me that my soul is flooded with peace while I wait upon You, for You alone are my salvation.

My Lord, I am tired physically, mentally, and emotionally; therefore, I release control and lean fully on Your faithfulness to lead me beside still waters so I can sleep tonight. Lord, there is so much noise out there, distractions, and many things to worry about. However, I thank you for the promise to rescue me from these concerns that can steal my sleep.

Thank you for being my refuge, my salvation, and my rest. I choose to trust in You completely knowing that as I sleep You are watching over me. May my soul find true peace in Your presence as I sleep tonight in Jesus' name. Amen.

31 Days to Overcoming Insomnia

JOURNAL
"Sound Sleep is Important"

Morning Cognitive Renewal Statements

- Today, I choose to surrender all control to God. I trust in His plans, and I rest in His peace. My soul finds true rest in Him, and I am renewed by His strength.
- I release all anxiety and tension to God. I trust Him with my day, and I walk forward in peace, knowing that my rest comes from Him.

Morning Journal Guided Reflections

What am I holding onto that I need to surrender to God today? How can I practice releasing control and trusting God with my plans and worries?

_____
_____
_____
_____
_____
_____
_____
_____
_____
_____
_____
_____
_____
_____
_____
_____

Morning Mindful Rest Practices

- **Surrendering Breath Prayer**
  Begin your day with 5 minutes of quiet breathing. As you inhale, say, *"I receive Your peace."* As you exhale, say, *"I surrender my worries."* Repeat this, allowing your body and mind to align with the act of surrender and trust in God.

- **Daily Release Meditation**
  Take a moment to identify one area of your life where you've been holding onto control. Write this down, then say aloud, *"God, I surrender this to You. I trust You with this part of my life."* Release that specific concern as you start your day.

Unlock Deep Sleep Secrets

Evening Cognitive Renewal Statements

- As I lay down to sleep, I surrender every worry and burden to God. I trust Him with all that concerns me, and I enter into His perfect rest.
- I release control over tomorrow and rest in God's care tonight. His peace surrounds me, and I trust Him to work as I sleep.

Evening Journal Guided Reflections

What burdens did I carry today that I need to surrender before bed?

_____
_____
_____
_____
_____
_____

How did surrendering to God throughout the day impact my peace and ability to rest?

_____
_____
_____
_____
_____
_____

Evening Mindful Rest Practices

- **Nightly Surrender**
  Before bed, sit quietly and think about the things that are weighing on your heart or causing stress. One by one, speak each concern aloud, followed by, *"I surrender this to You, Lord."* Feel the weight lift as you release each burden, trusting God to handle them.

- **Psalm 62 Reflection**
  Slowly read Psalm 62:1 before bed. Reflect on the truth that rest comes from God alone. Let His peace wash over you as you meditate on this verse. Say aloud, *"I find rest in You, God,"* and allow this affirmation to calm your mind and prepare you for peaceful sleep.

31 Days to Overcoming Insomnia

Weekly Reflection
Reflect on how surrendering control has affected your sleep and overall sense of peace this week. What areas of your life have been easier to let go of, and where do you still need to trust God more?

_____
_____
_____
_____
_____
_____
_____

"Surrender and Rest" In Practice
Surrendering is an active process that invites you to place your trust in God and release the things you can't control. Through morning and evening practices of surrender, you create space for God's peace to replace anxiety, which leads to deeper rest and sound sleep. Letting go of control allows God to work in your life and brings you into a place of stillness, where true rest is found.

Day 20
UNWINDING – FINDING PEACE IN THE STILLNESS

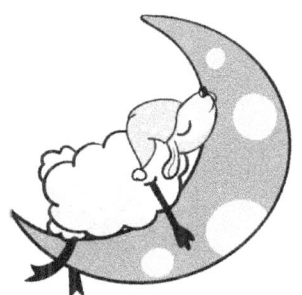

Psalm 23:2 (NIV):
"He makes me lie down in green pastures, he leads me beside quiet waters."

In today's hectic society, downtime is a rare and precious gift. The buzz of technology, the pressures of work and family, the demands to always be "on," is so insufferable that there is no room for rest. Our heads are usually overworked, our bodies needing rest by the time evening rolls around. But it doesn't help that no matter how worn we are, sleep is just not there because we can't rest.

To unwind is not about switching off the lights and hoping for the best. It's the conscious release of all that stress, anxiety, worry and stress that was in your body throughout the day. It's letting go, shutting down the voice, and handing it over to tranquility. The good news is, there's an easy road to actual relaxation, and that road is straight to good sleep.

And the answer to that is ancient, but timeless wisdom: Psalm 23:2: *"He makes me lie down in green pastures, he leads me beside still waters."*

This is the saying of relaxation, this poem. It conjures a picture of tranquility, silence, rest. But God has an oasis, in the middle of all the noise in the world, where we can lay down our worries and be restful. The "green pastures" are where the body can be fed, and the "still waters" are where the peace can flow in our thoughts. It's an image of recharging in its purest form, of sitting back, letting ourselves in and letting go.

The Struggle to Unwind
Relaxation isn't always so easy. The more we attempt to forget the day, the less we can settle down. Our minds keep going round and round in our heads—about things we still need to

31 Days to Overcoming Insomnia

get done, about tomorrow, or how sad we feel at the end of the day. We don't know how to sleep; it's like our brains are a different animal. But the reality is: Relaxing is a decision and it's deliberate.

Psalm 23:2 teaches us the call to give up and lie down. As the line "He makes me lie down" hints, rest isn't just passive. It takes an act of turning a corner— of becoming still. Yet with so much in our life to keep us awake, what do we do when it's time to relax? How can we be unworried enough to enjoy the rest promised in Psalm 23?

The Power of Stillness

And not only that: quietness doesn't mean there is nothing to do but there is silence. It's there, in the silence, that you first rest. Psalm 23:22-23 The "still waters" stand for an oasis of peace and refreshment in the heart. Let's say you're standing on the bank of a still lake and the waves calm your mind. That is what stillness is, the quiet that makes us whole from within.

And when it comes to sleep, stillness is the state of mind and emotion we must enter to fully unwind. This starts with letting go of the day's burden in your mind. When you stop thinking about things, even for a few minutes, you are granting your unconscious permission to sleep. Not by letting go of your obligations, but by choosing to unwind them for the time being so your brain and body can recharge.

Unwinding Through Psalm 23:2

We are given a road map to rest in Psalm 23:2. It is about literally leading ourselves to a place of stillness. So how can we take this verse to bed to relax and rewind, and get a good night's sleep?

> ### *Leave the Day's Pressure Behind*
> You can't relax without first recognizing how tired you are. Our days are full, where we can be piled up from work, love, or simply our inner world. Psalm 23:2 says, *"He makes me lie down in green pastures."* Notice the word "makes." This isn't passive; it's intentional. Unwinding sometimes means you have to "cease" yourself. And you need to take a chance to let the day go.
>
> One of the exercises can be done before going to sleep: scan every single part of your body and unwind gently. Beginning with your toes, reach up to your head, trying not to tighten or itch. You release the tension in your body and then you open the doors to mental and emotional calm.
>
> ### *Breathe and Center Your Mind*
> If we want to relax, we have to settle—both mentally and physically. Breath is a really good medicine for calming the mind and body. Pause to notice the breath: deep, long

Unlock Deep Sleep Secrets

inhale, and long, gentle exhale. Breathe in with your heart—picture the air filling you with tranquility, and as you exhale, release any stress, worry, or thoughts of anxiety.

While breathing, imagine the "still waters" of Psalm 23. Imagine you're by a still lake, listening to the gentle eddy of the waves. Let this picture be in your head, the one you use as a symbol—calm, clear, untroubled. You know, let's say your thoughts are quieter as you breathe, and your brain is still. This technique is not only a stress-busting activity, but it also communicates to your unconscious that it is time to relax and get ready for sleep.

Create a Sleepy Nighttime Habit
There is no de-stressing better than setting a soothing bedtime routine. Psalm 23:2 equates sleeping in a green field with resting and abandonment. Like the sheep who goes to sleep in the field, you too must establish the right environment for rest.

Build a soothing pre-sleep ritual—read a book, meditate, or play relaxing music. Don't do things that overstimulate your brain, such as composing emails, surfing the internet, or having emotional conversations. Rather, do things that signal to your body and brain that the day is over and it's time to get some sleep.

Give Up Power and Let Peace Take Over
And the final stage of unwinding is relinquishing power. Psalm 23:2 presents the picture of quiet, sure submission. To sit in pastures and huddle next to still water is a picture of total trust. Likewise, when you're relaxing, you must believe it will be all right. All the day's anxieties, the things you haven't completed, the future's unknowns, those can wait. Until you can give yourself a rest, for now.

Among the best ways to relax is to pray or meditate and put your concerns and ideas before God. Even a simple prayer such as, *"I let go and know I'm secure, that I'm at ease, and that I'm ready to go to sleep,"* will communicate to your unconscious that it's time to surrender. When you stop trying to be in charge, you free yourself up for sleep.

Why Getting Rid of Yourself is Crucial to Sleeping Well
Relaxation is not only about physical rest—it is also about psychological and emotional surrender. The real rest is when you let yourself go and believe everything is OK. By actually letting go, you leave time for sound sleep, without worry and stress.

As I always tell people, it's not laying on your back that is in Psalm 23:2 – it's reclining into silence. It's a reminder to quiet your brain, let go of the worries of the day, believe in the silence of stillness.

This evening, before you head to bed, release the mental clutter and be still. Just as pastures

31 Days to Overcoming Insomnia

and still waters soothe the spirit, so let yourself sit and sooth in the quiet before bedtime. And there you'll sleep, soul and body.

Unwind with intention. Trust in the stillness. So put your mind and body at rest with the quiet of Psalm 23. The night is on the way.

Prayer for the Journey

Dear God, as I prepare to sleep this evening, I come before You humbly seeking Your help to achieve sweet sleep. I thank You for being my Good Shepherd, the One who leads me into peace and rest. Thank you for the promise You gave me in Psalms 23:2, that You continuously make me lie down in green pastures and lead me beside still waters.

Tonight, I look forward to green pastures of restful sleep and green pastures of security. Just as sheep only lie down when they feel safe, full and free from fear, so do I decree, I feel safe in the Lord's arms. I am full of peace and free from anxiety. I acknowledge that You are the One who provides spiritual nourishment and true rest. Thank you for the still waters that are flooding my soul tonight. I decree there are no rushing waters that create panic and disturb my sweet sleep. I realize that You are the only one who authentically calms my soul and provides refreshment.

I decree that Your presence is now surrounding me like soft green pastures, comforting and calming me. I speak peace to unsetting thoughts, peace to my anxious heart. Your peace is washing over me like gentle waters.

I decree, that tonight, I will sleep soundly, undisturbed by all cares because your peace envelops me. Thank You for Your faithfulness and loving care, which sustain me through each moment. Just as a shepherd protects and care for his sheep, I trust You are watching over me as I sleep. In Jesus' name. Amen.

Unlock Deep Sleep Secrets

JOURNAL
"Sound Sleep is Important"

Morning Cognitive Renewal Statements

- As I begin my day, I carry the peace within me. I release all prolonged pressure and accept calm. I am grounded in God's peacefulness, and I face today with a clear, peaceful mind.

Morning Journal Guided Reflections

How can I invite peace and calm into my day today? What actions or thoughts will help me stay in a place of rest, even when faced with stress?

_____
_____
_____
_____
_____
_____
_____
_____
_____
_____
_____
_____
_____
_____
_____
_____

Evening Cognitive Renewal Statements

- This evening, I release all my worries and tension. I relinquish what no longer serves me and welcome peace. My mind is relaxed, my body is stress-free, and I trust God's rest to renew me for tomorrow."

Evening Journal Guided Reflections

- Imagine you are turning off a switch, letting go of all the day's energy and stress. What is one thing you achieved today that you're proud of? Celebrate it and release anything that no longer serves you. Now, visualize yourself being revived, filled with peace, ready to sleep deeply and wake up renewed.

31 Days to Overcoming Insomnia

Evening Mindful Rest Practices

- **Unwind with Quiet Reflection**
  Take 5-10 minutes before bed to sit in silence or with soft music. Close your eyes and picture the quiet waters from Psalm 23:2. Imagine yourself by a serene stream, letting the water carry away any lingering stress or thoughts. As you breathe deeply, repeat, *"He leads me beside quiet waters."*
- **Light Stretching Routine**
  Perform a gentle stretching routine that focuses on releasing tension in your muscles. Each stretch should be slow and calming, helping your body to relax. As you stretch, repeat a calming verse or affirmation, such as, *"God's peace surrounds me."*

Weekly Reflection

How did I experience God's peace today? In what ways did He lead me beside quiet waters? How has intentional unwinding each night affected the quality of my sleep and overall sense of peace? Where do I still need to release control or tension?

_____
_____
_____
_____
_____
_____
_____
_____
_____
_____
_____
_____
_____
_____
_____
_____
_____
_____

"Unwinding" in Practice

Unwinding is an intentional act of surrendering to God's peace, allowing His presence to restore your mind, body, and spirit. By incorporating quiet moments of reflection, stretching, and calming affirmations, you create a space for peace to replace tension, enabling your body to rest deeply in God's care. This practice fosters a rhythm of peace that not only prepares you for restful sleep. but also helps you carry calmness into your daily life.

Day 21
THE IMPORTANCE OF DOWNTIME FOR MENTAL HEALTH

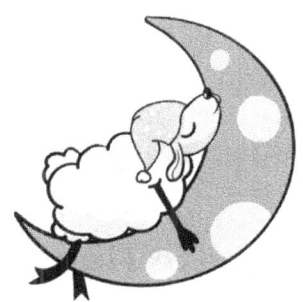

Exodus 20:8:10 (NIV):
"Remember the Sabbath day, to keep it holy. Six days you shall labor, and do all your work, but the seventh day is a Sabbath to the Lord your God. On it, you shall not do any work."

It's a world where, with all the demands and to-dos going on, we can never take a breath, stop, or even take a shower. We're all on the go, working, dating, and other commitments. But with all that, we can get lost, psychologically drained, and emotionally drained. We cannot stress enough the mental health significance of downtime.

"But I don't have time for sleep. I gotta keep going, keep making, keep succeeding!" Except that you don't intentionally take time off, your mind, body, and soul burn.

God Himself commands us with a very powerful command in Exodus 20:8-10–rest. He has set aside a day off, a "Sabbath" in which we are away from our work and can just be. The sage ship of God in this command was not just for the Israelites: it's for us, too. Pause, ponder, and recharge are important mental practices.

Let's dive in to see why unwinding is not a luxury; it's necessary. And if we value rest, then we are clearer, more productive, and calmer.

God's Design for Rest
God tells His people in Exodus 20:8-10 to allow one day a week to be a resting day. It wasn't just a recommendation; it was a script from God for mental, emotional, and physical

31 Days to Overcoming Insomnia

health. Remember the Sabbath day and keep it holy. This is not just religious discipline. It is a profound rule God put in place for our spiritual health.

God also recognized that His children would have to rest more than they slept for their function to be as good as possible. They needed to get their heads and hearts back on top. The Sabbath was a day when they could take a break from work and to do something that revived their spirits. It was not a day of productivity or to-do lists. It was a day of solitude, prayer, communion, and rest.

Mental health requires intentional breaks. Our minds also need sleep to cope with emotions, thoughts, and stressors, like our bodies do. When we can see that there are times of no activity, we allow ourselves to reset. We burn out and become emotionally depleted if we're always on the job. But if we spend our time in the rest, then we are better prepared for the future.

The Health Benefits of Restorative Time for the Mind

But why does this downtime matter so much to our mental health? But what if we rest, as God in Exodus 20:8-10 tells us to?

> ***Downtime Resets Our Brains and Our Muscles:*** We get information, stress, and a new head when we rest often enough. We do so because we need energy from rest. We're mentally, emotionally and otherwise mentally exhausted.
>
> ***Downtime Reduces Stress and Anxiety:*** Stress and anxiety are the scourge of the mind. It affects our mood, our choices, and even our bodies. Rest and unplugging from everyday work help our nervous system relax. It provides us with time to breathe, think, and rest in the middle of the storm. When we actively schedule pauses, we manage the stresses in our life, which are not good for our psyche.
>
> ***Downtime Improves Focus and Productivity:*** Despite the contrary, taking breaks is actually more productive. When we train all the time and don't rest, we lose focus. Our brains get fuzzy and our creative thinking decreases. Yet when we celebrate rest, our mind functions better, and we can concentrate better when we are back in the office. It's not that we spend the day off doing nothing; it's about recharging our capacity to do more.
>
> ***Downtime Increases Emotional Health:*** We need to get into touch with feelings and sensations we might otherwise never have the chance to discuss. If we don't get enough rest, we're emotionally exhausted, burned out, irritable, and even depressed. To pause and think is to gain perspective, let go, and come back to ourselves. When we allow ourselves to rest, we make room for psychological restoration.

Unlock Deep Sleep Secrets

Prayer for the Journey

Dear God, thank you for the blessing of rest. It's a time You have set aside for me to be regenerated and renewed. You went as far as establishing the Sabbath as a reminder that I do not have to strive endlessly, but I can trust in Your provisions and care. Tonight, I surrender my burdens and worries into Your hands being fully convinced that You desire me to have sweet sleep.

You have established a rhythm of work followed by rest. It is Your will that I have restful sleep, so let Your will be done in my life tonight. Rest is not just a luxury but a divine principle. It's Your design for my well-being, so I embrace this principle tonight. My mind and body require time to heal from the pressures and demands of my daily life. Thank you for ordaining this night for the supernatural replenishing of my body, soul, and spirit.

Lord, as I lay my head down to sleep tonight, I know Your plans for me are good so I trust You with all that concerns me. I decree that in the morning, I will wake up strengthened and refreshed, ready to continue walking in Your purpose for my life. Thank you for feeling me with peace as I sleep, for being my refuge and watching over me in Jesus' name. Amen.

31 Days to Overcoming Insomnia

JOURNAL
"Sound Sleep is Important"

Morning Cognitive Renewal Statements

- I embrace the importance of downtime for my mental health.
- I am deserving of rest and rejuvenation.
- Today, I will prioritize my well-being and take mindful breaks.

Morning Journal Guided Reflections

What are three things I can do today to prioritize my downtime?

_____
_____
_____
_____
_____

How can I incorporate moments of calm into my busy schedule?

_____
_____
_____
_____
_____

Morning Mindful Rest Practices

- **Gentle Stretching:** Spend 10 minutes doing light stretches to awaken your body and release tension.
- **Mindful Breathing:** Practice deep breathing for a few minutes to set a calm tone for the day ahead.
- **Nature Walk:** Take a short walk outdoors to enjoy the fresh air and connect with nature.

Evening Cognitive Renewal Statements

- I release the stress of the day and welcome peace into my mind.
- I honor my body by allowing it to rest and restore.
- Each moment of downtime enriches my life and enhances my sleep.

Unlock Deep Sleep Secrets

Evening Journal Guided Reflections

Did I take enough time for myself today?

_____
_____
_____
_____
_____

What helped me relax?

_____
_____
_____
_____
_____
_____

How did my downtime impact my mood and overall well-being?

_____
_____
_____
_____
_____
_____

Evening Mindful Rest Practices

- **Relaxing Yoga:** Engage in a gentle yoga session in the evening to unwind and prepare for sleep.

- **Journaling:** Write about your day, focusing on moments of gratitude and relaxation.

    _____
    _____
    _____
    _____
    _____
    _____
    _____

- **Reading:** Spend 20-30 minutes reading a book that inspires or calms you before bed.

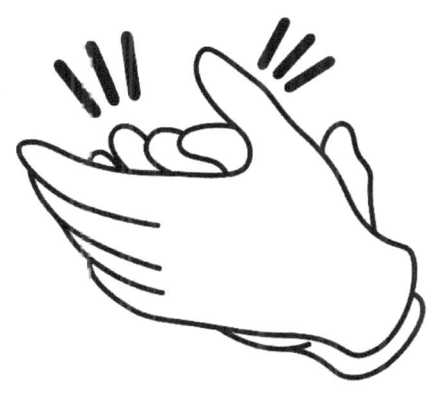

**WAY TO GO!!!
YOU MADE IT THROUGH
21 DAYS OF SLEEP REJUVENATION!**

Day 22
BE CONNECTED TO THE SECRET PLACE

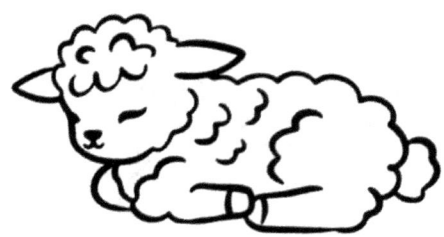

Psalm 91:1 (NIV):
"He who dwells in the shelter of the Most High will rest in the shadow of the Almighty."

The Power of the Secret Place
In a world that pushes us in various directions all the time, we're ill-balanced, nervous, or overworked. The din of existence, work, friendships, and obligations can obliterate the silence to thrive. Yet something powerful is on the horizon for Psalm 91:1 that promises to be more than this, something revolutionary. It is a call to live under the cover of the One Who is high—to stay down and sleep under the awning of the Great One.

This tucked-away space, where God is most felt, is not a place; it's a spiritual sanctuary where we are in real contact with God. It is where the world stops making noise, and we get the rest and tranquility only God can offer.

Experiencing the secret is not a cult; it is a way to rest, to heal, to get on top of life's storms. So, let's find out in what it is to be in God's presence, how to enter the inner realm, and how keeping in contact with it changes everything.

Understanding the Secret Place
This secret is where God is most present. It's not somewhere we must go there, but it's a heart position. Psalm 91:1 calls it a "shelter" and "shadow," which are descriptions of security, comfort, and intimacy. To live in the protection of the Most High is to live in God—not going to God when we are in need of help, but living in His presence, sleeping under His cover, coming into refuge in Him every single day.

Psalm 91:1 implies that to dwell is a continuous connection. It's being a relationship with God so intimate that His presence is natural territory. Suppose you have God's wisdom,

Unlock Deep Sleep Secrets

peace, and power in your fingertips all the time—when you are at work, when you are at home, when things get tough. That is the force of living enmeshed in hidden space.

The Secret Place: A Resting Place

Life is so stressful, difficult, and busy. But if we are attached to the secret site, we are put to rest. Psalm 91:1 says they will sleep in the shadow of God when they are under His protection. This rest isn't just physical, but it's intellectual and spiritual, too. And there we find the peace we so long for.

The secret place of rest is not the abandonment of work and movement. That's peace in a storm. It's knowing that even in the craziest or hardest times, we're still saved and provided for by the God of heaven. We are living from security, not tension, because of this connection. So, here is what rest looks like in the secret place:

Mental rest: In God's presence, your mind, which is stuffed with anxieties and anxieties, is at rest.

Spiritual rest: Your heart, tormented by the things of this world, is restorative with the presence of God. Your soul, hungry for meaning and purpose, is renewed in God's wisdom eternal.

And this sleep comes because you know that God takes care of you no matter what happens. If you are connected to the hidden place, you're connected to peace that guards your heart and mind all the time.

The Secret Place: A Sanctuary of Safety

In Psalm 91:1, God's protection is called the "shadow of the Almighty." A shadow was a type of covering and shielding in the Old Testament. Suppose you were under the shadow of the strongest power in the universe—the God of all powers. This isn't just a sidekick; this is a safe place.

When you are linked to the secret place, no matter how stormy the world around you gets, you are covered with the protection of God. That doesn't mean there won't be some things in life that you experience hardships. It just means that in the midst of those hardships God will be with you.

So if there is a terror, you are safe. You are protected when the going gets tough. When the unknown is near, you know that the Most High is your castle. To live in the secret place is to live in the safest house. God's armor shields you from the evils that would devour your brain, heart, and soul.

31 Days to Overcoming Insomnia

How to Be Linked to the Secret Place
To be connected to the hidden place is a daily decision. These are concrete steps to keep you connected to God, where you'll be able to sleep, be secure, and rest.

- **Daily Prayer/Meditation: Establish Time Daily**
  The secret place is not one you happen upon by accident—it's the one you cultivate through intentional time with God. Take the time to pray and ponder Scripture each morning. Take Psalm 91:1 as your anchor because you will be able to be in the presence of God anywhere you are.

  - **Exercise:** Take 10-15 minutes in the morning to sit quietly, meditate on God's Word, and speak to God from your heart. Invite Him into your day.

- **Embrace Stillness and Solitude**
  You can get distracted in your life by living—moving and then never notice that you're still. But the secret is found when there is nothing else to do. Jesus would retreat to prayerful places; so, you can also carve out time in your day to just sit there with God.

  - **Exercise:** Recess at the beginning of the day—go outside, go to a dark room, sit with your eyes closed for 10 minutes. Let God's presence surround you.

- **Cultivate a Heart of Trust**
  The hidden room is the place where we surrender all to God without worries and fears. The more we come to believe God, the more we get to know His sanctum. Your house is made from trust. Rely on Him to save, teach, and supply.

  - **Exercise:** Pause in the middle of worry or fear and really sit with your breathing. Declare that you trust in God and that He is your refuge.

- **Practice Gratitude**
  The practice of Thanksgiving serves as a powerful means to remain connected to the secret place through the cultivation of gratitude. God is what we lack. Expressing thanks to Him for His presence, along with His safety and stillness, will open the door further to enable His work.

Prayer for the Journey
Dear God, as I lay down to sleep tonight, I want to thank you for the promise You made in Psalms 91:1, a psalm of refuge, because I need refuge from sleeplessness. Yes, Lord, I need protection from a restless mind and an unstable heart. Show me how to dwell in Your

Unlock Deep Sleep Secrets

secret place. I want to stay near to You because it's Your presence that provides peace safety and rest.

Let Your presence fill this room, for Your presence provides the ultimate shelter and peace. I position myself under Your divine covering far from lingering disturbing and distressing thoughts. I now command fear, anxious thoughts, and every worry that try to steal my rest to leave me now. I am not alone; God is for me.

I decree You are my refuge, fortress, and resting place. I totally trust You, because I know You are watching over me. You never slumber nor sleep; You are my guardian, God. Thank you for being my protector and for giving me the gift of sleep. I am confident in Your unfailing love and rest in You tonight in Jesus's name. Amen.

31 Days to Overcoming Insomnia

JOURNAL
"Sound Sleep is Important"

Morning Cognitive Renewal Statements

- I dwell in the secret place of the Most-High where I find safety and peace.
- Today, I open my heart to God's presence and guidance.
- I am worthy of rest and connection with God.

Morning Journal Guided Reflections

What plans can I set today to prioritize my time in the secret place?

_____
_____
_____
_____
_____

How can I cultivate an attitude of openness and receptivity to God's presence today?

_____
_____
_____
_____
_____

Morning Mindful Rest Practices

Quiet Time for Reflection: Spend 10-15 minutes in silence, focusing on your breath. Visualize yourself entering the secret place, feeling God's presence envelop you.

Scripture Meditation: Read and meditate on Psalm 91. Write down any thoughts or feelings that arise and how they resonate with your current life situation.

_____
_____
_____
_____
_____
_____
_____

Unlock Deep Sleep Secrets

Nature Connection: Go for a short walk outside. Use this time to appreciate creation, pray, and converse with God, inviting His presence into your day.

Evening Cognitive Renewal Statements

- I release the cares of the day and rest in God's embrace.
- My time in the secret place renews my spirit and strengthens my faith.
- I trust that God's peace surrounds me as I prepare for restful sleep.

Evening Journal Guided Reflections

Did I spend time in the secret place today? _____

What did I experience or feel? What insights or comfort did I gain from my connection with God? How can I carry that into tomorrow?

_____
_____
_____
_____
_____
_____
_____

Evening Mindful Rest Practice

Gratitude Journaling: Write down three things you are grateful for from your day. Reflect on how God has been present in those moments, fostering a sense of connection and thankfulness.

- I am grateful for _____
- I am thankful for _____
- I appreciate for _____

Guided Prayer: Spend 10-15 minutes in prayer, focusing on surrendering any worries or stresses. Use this time to listen for God's voice and invite His peace into your heart.

Relaxing Yoga or Stretching: Engage in gentle stretching or a restorative yoga practice to relax your body and prepare for sleep, inviting a sense of calm and peace.

Day 23
SLEEP-FRIENDLY FOODS: WHAT TO EAT FOR BETTER ZZZS

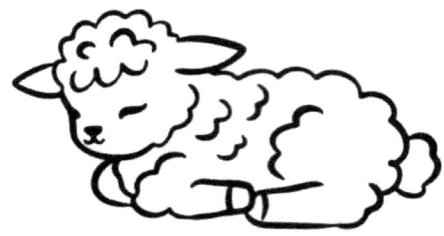

1 Corinthians 10:31 (NIV):
"So whether you eat or drink or whatever you do, do it all for the glory of God."

The Relationship Between Food and Sleep

We all know that a decent night's sleep is essential for general well-being. But what if the key to better sleep is in your kitchen? We think about things like getting into bed at a certain time or having the ideal sleeping situation, but your diet also affects your sleep.

We're reminded in Psalm 127:2 that God is so good that He gives us sleep. Yet we can all take care of our bodies and brains—and feed them the right kind of food for restful, reviving sleep. Here's a sleep-friendly food guide for your comfort to get you asleep fast and through the night.

The Truth About the Science of Sleep and Food

Before we dive into the best sleep foods, let's take a short peek at why food impacts sleep. Some foods contain nutrients that keep our sleep-wake cycles stable and our sleeping patterns better. Such nutrients can also affect levels of melatonin and serotonin, two sleep hormones.

Melatonin is the "sleep hormone" because it is your body's internal clock telling your brain it's time to fall asleep. Serotonin (the "feel-good" neurotransmitter) can be turned into melatonin by the body, making it conducive to sleep. When you include a few sleep-promoting foods in your diet, it's easy to naturally increase the production of these hormones and be able to fall and stay asleep.

Unlock Deep Sleep Secrets

Top Sleep-Friendly Foods
Here are some foods that aid in sleeping so your body gets all the nutrition for a restful night.

Almonds: A Magnesium Powerhouse
Magnesium is a mineral that's involved in sleeping by helping your muscles relax and your nervous system calm down. Almonds are packed with magnesium, so they can increase the quality and length of your sleep.

How to enjoy: Drink a cup of tea and have a handful of almonds before bed. Pour almond butter on a piece of wholegrain toast for a nighttime snack.

Cherries: Natural Source of Melatonin
Cherries (especially tart cherries) are among the very few natural foods rich in melatonin, the hormone that sets your sleep cycle. Drink some tart cherry juice or have a small handful of fresh cherries in the evening, and you'll get a better sleep.

How to enjoy: Drink a small glass of tart cherry juice before bed. Enjoy a bowl of fresh cherries or dried cherries as a pre-sleep snack.

Bananas: A Potassium-Rich Snack
Bananas are also rich in potassium, which calms the muscles and nerves. You also get tryptophan, an amino acid your body uses to produce serotonin and melatonin, the sleep hormones.

How to enjoy: Slice up a banana and layer it over your morning oatmeal or eat one in bed. Serve with some almonds to make a magnesium-tryptophan power combo!

Oats: A Cozy, Sleep-Inducing Carbohydrate
Oats contain melatonin and complex carbs, both of which boost serotonin. All of this means oats are an ideal sleep-inducing food to keep you powered up for the long haul, but without waking you up.

How to enjoy: Serve oatmeal with some cinnamon in the morning before going to bed. Prepare overnight oats for an easy healthy snack before bed.

Herbal Teas: Chamomile and Lavender
Herbal teas are centuries-old and help with relaxation and sleeping. Chamomile is especially good for calming: an antioxidant called apigenin binds to certain receptors in the brain, making us sleepy. Lavender has a calming fragrance that can help with anxiety and sleep quality.

How to enjoy: Drink a cup of chamomile or lavender tea 30 minutes before bed. Serve with some honey for sweetness and rest.

31 Days to Overcoming Insomnia

Kiwi: A Sleep Superfood
Kiwis are brimming with antioxidants, vitamins, and serotonin-promoting compounds. Research has shown that kiwi before bed increases sleep quality, reduces the time it takes for you to go to sleep, and prolongs sleep.

How to enjoy: Eat 2 kiwis about an hour before bed to help you get to sleep. Try them in your nocturnal smoothie or alongside some nuts.

Turkey: A Tryptophan Boost
Turkey can be one of the groggiest foods after Thanksgiving dinner, and for good reason! It's packed with tryptophan, an amino acid that helps the body create serotonin and melatonin to relax and sleep.

How to enjoy: Snack on a little turkey sandwich on whole grain bread in the evening. Serve some turkey salad with a few greens for dinner.

Spinach and Leafy Greens: Magnesium and Folate
Spinach, kale, and Swiss chard are high in magnesium and folate, which help your body settle down and get ready for bed. Magnesium maintains melatonin and folate soothes anxiety and stress.

How to enjoy: Include spinach in your nightly salad or smoothie. Fry up some kale or Swiss chard for dinner.

Foods to Avoid Before Bed
You get good sleep with some foods and poor sleep with others. Here are a few things you can stay away from during those final hours before bed:

- *Caffeine:* In coffee, tea, chocolate and certain beverages, caffeine is a waking agent. Avoid caffeine at least 6 hours before going to sleep.

- *Fats and heavy meals:* A high-fat diet such as fried foods or greasy snacks will give you indigestion and discomfort, which could interfere with sleep.

- *Sweets:* Adding sugar to snacks is a high-sugar recipe for a spike in your blood sugar that will set you up for an energy hit that will keep you awake.

- *Hot food:* Hot foods make your body warm and makes you feel dizzy, which disturbs your sleep.

Unlock Deep Sleep Secrets

Creating a Sleep-Friendly Evening Routine
Now that we know what foods are sleep-promoting, how can we start eating them every day to experience more ZZZ's? For a sleep-friendly night, here are a few ideas:

- *Plan Your Evening Meals*
  Eat a light, sleep-friendly dinner later in the day. Pick foods with tryptophan (turkey or bananas), magnesium (almonds or spinach), and melatonin (cherries or oats). Don't eat big meals or foods that are hot close to bedtime.

- *Create a Bedtime Snack Ritual*
  Then about an hour before bed, have a little snack that has sleep-friendly foods in it. It can be as healing as an almond butter banana or a warm glass of chamomile tea.

- *Hydrate, But Not Too Much*
  Water throughout the day is good, but don't drink a ton of water just before going to sleep to save yourself from having to wake up in the middle of the night to go bathroom.

- *Create a Relaxing Atmosphere*
  Add a twilight space, music, or aromatherapy to go along with your sleep foods. Designing a quiet space is telling your body it's time to relax and rest.

Sleep Starts with Eating Well
God is so good to give us rest, as we're told in Psalm 127:2. But to get the right kind of restful sleep, we have to feed our bodies well, too. When you put foods that promote sleep, such as almonds, cherries, and bananas in your nightly diet, you will get a better night's rest and wake up refreshed and full of energy.

Don't forget that healthy food doesn't only nourish your body, but it is good for your mental and emotional health, too. So, next time you are gearing up for a good night's sleep, eat things that will relax your body and brain and let you get some well-deserved shut-eye. Sleep tight and may your ZZZs be one of peace and refreshment!

Prayer for the Journey
Dear God, as I get ready to settle in tonight, I thank you for the gift of life. Thank you for the reminder You issued in 1 Corinthians 10:31, that everything I do, even the simple act of sleeping, should be done for Your glory. Consequently, tonight I surrender my thoughts, my body, and my heart – my entire being to You.

Dad, I have a humble request. Can You please help me to live my life honoring You even through food? You see, I am aware that the way I eat can have devastating consequences

31 Days to Overcoming Insomnia

in the pursuit of satisfying rest. Help me to choose foods that promote sweet sleep, hence bringing peace, restoration, and equilibrium in my body, which is Your temple.
Help me to be constantly aware of how I spend my time and energy because I want to make choices that always bring glory to You. I now receive Your peace that surpasses all understanding. I rest in the shadow of Your love because I put my trust in You.
I lay down any feeling of shame about my previous actions and I receive the purification of my mind and body now. Help me stay more connected to You since You hold the script for my life.

I decree I receive from the fulness of the sleep Jesus had on that rocky boat, and of the fulness of Your power and knowledge to make good decisions that will bring me good sleep. As I lay my head on my pillow, I decree You are the source of sleep from which I have receive, so that my body might be restored, my mind stilled, and my soul at be peace. In the matchless name of King Jesus. Amen.

Unlock Deep Sleep Secrets

JOURNAL
"Sound Sleep is Important"

Morning Cognitive Renewal Statements

- I honor God with my food choices, nourishing my body for optimal health.
- Today, I choose foods that promote restful sleep and rejuvenation.
- I am grateful for the abundance of nutritious options available to me.

Morning Journal Guided Reflections

What nutritious foods can I include in my meals today to support better sleep?

_____
_____
_____
_____

How can I plan my meals to avoid heavy or spicy foods close to bedtime?

_____
_____
_____
_____

Morning Mindful Rest Practices

- **Plan Your Meals:** Take 10 minutes to create a meal plan for the day, incorporating sleep-friendly foods, such as whole grains, leafy greens, nuts, seeds, and lean proteins.
- **Create a Grocery List:** Make a list of sleep-promoting foods to buy this week, focusing on items like bananas, oats, chamomile tea, and fish rich in omega-3 fatty acids.
- **Hydration Reminder:** Start your day with a glass of water. Consider adding a slice of lemon or cucumber for flavor, keeping hydration in mind.

Evening Cognitive Renewal Statements

- I release any stress from the day and prepare my body for peaceful sleep.
- The foods I consumed today support my well-being and restfulness.
- I trust that my body knows how to rejuvenate and restore itself.

31 Days to Overcoming Insomnia

Evening Guided Reflections

Did I make sleep-friendly food choices today? _____

How did they affect my energy and mood? What were my thoughts and feelings around my eating habits today, and how can I improve tomorrow?

_____
_____
_____
_____
_____
_____
_____
_____

Evening Mindful Rest Practices

- **Relaxing Herbal Tea:** Brew a cup of chamomile or valerian root tea before bed. Spend 10 minutes enjoying this calming drink while reflecting on your day.
- **Mindful Eating:** Prepare a light evening snack, such as yogurt with honey and walnuts or a small bowl of oatmeal. Eat slowly and savor each bite, focusing on the flavors and textures.

Reflection Journal: Spend 5-10 minutes writing about how your food choices influenced your day, particularly regarding your energy levels and mood.

Day 24
FROM PAIN TO PEACE: NAVIGATING SLEEP AFTER TRAUMA

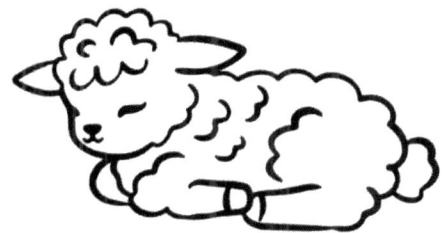

Psalm 147:3 (NIV):
"He heals the brokenhearted and binds up their wounds."

Jeremiah 29:11 (NIV):
"For I know the plans I have for you," declares the Lord, "plans to prosper you and not to harm you, plans to give you hope and a future."

The world, as you know, moves under your feet when trauma happens. Your brain runs through red tape, scares, and questions. Here is where that most impossible thing we're always looking for turns into something we all need most: sleep. You could be lying in bed, the world crushing you, and you can't sleep.

Sleep, that organic, survival activity, is now a battlefield. You cannot fall asleep because the trauma is so fresh, too heavy, for you to sleep. You have your brain on a whirlwind, replaying the trauma, your heart fatigued to rest. But what if God's gift is not the sum of one night alone? But what if you could get peace and sleep, right when you're at your most depressed?

We read in Psalm 147:3 that God is doing what it takes to restore the lost. He is stitching the scabs that haunt us, that hurt our hearts, and that deprive us of serenity. And Jeremiah 29:11 tells us that God's got our future figured out— plans of health not disease, plans of redemption. He does not leave it only in the heart— He touches all areas of our being, even our sleep.

This is not the day where trauma is denied or healing is rushed. Instead, it's walking from hurt to joy, believing God has a plan for you, and that His joy can settle the storm in your heart so that you can fall asleep in Him.

31 Days to Overcoming Insomnia

The Traumatic Imprint on Sleep
Trauma does profound things, and it often changes the way we see life unexpectedly. Perhaps the most important, and immediate, consequence is that of sleeping.

There are also those for whom rest simply isn't an option after a nightmare. The body is hyperarousal all the time, the "fight or flight" response going on well past bedtime. You don't sleep because your brain is processing, still responding to the trauma that occurred.

Sleeplessness, nightmares, niggling thoughts, and hypervigilance break the sleep cycle so you feel tired but unable to sleep. It seems too far away to go to sleep, the deep sleep your body needs to repair and regenerate. And in the midst of this upheaval, Psalm 147:3 tells us to recite in song: God heals the brokenhearted and binds up our wounds. He is the one who feels the agony, the nightmares, the battles. There is a cure, and rest is that cure. Yet healing notwithstanding, trauma-relief takes intention. God is working His healing forces, but we must also have room for His stillness, not just for our healing souls, but also for our rest.

Navigating the Road from Pain to Peace
Traumatic recovery is a process, and it's one that we must wait for, trust in, and be prepared to let go of our hurts before God. But the beautiful thing about both Psalm 147:3 and Jeremiah 29:11 is that God has a plan for us, a plan that includes rest. His intention for us is not harm, but a promise and a future, a future that involves recovery and, yes, rest. Let's take a look at what it is we can do to go from pain to joy and give God our every moment:

- ***Acknowledge the Struggle, Let God In***
  The first thing you can do to recover is acknowledge it. Trauma can't be removed if we deny or conceal it. We do this far too often, but we think that by repressing the pain, it will go away. But the reality is that we heal best when we go right in and let God walk alongside us in the brokenness.

  We are told in Psalm 147:3 that God rescues the broken-hearted—He doesn't flee from what hurts. He is available to receive us in the wreck of our feelings, soothe us, and set us aright.

  <u>Mindful Rest Practices:</u> Before going to sleep, stop and think about the day and how hurt you have been. Speak it or type it, giving it over to God. Allow Him to come and redeem you.

  <u>Cognitive Renewal Statements:</u> I admit that I am hurt and ask God to put a patch on my heart. I open myself to His quiet in my life and in my sleep.

Unlock Deep Sleep Secrets

- ***Give Up Command and Lean on God's Design***
  Trauma is the most painful thing of all because it can leave us feeling powerless. We need solutions. We want it to be otherwise, and we want it to be made right. But the road from affliction to happiness is not a matter of us defining our situation, but it is us putting it in God's hands.

  We're reminded in Jeremiah 29:11 that God has a plan for us, and it is a hopeful plan with a future. God is in the background, orchestrating healing, even while we're going through trauma. We aren't to tamper with it, but to trust God is sovereign, and His will for us is tranquil.

  Mindful Rest Practices: Spend a few minutes before bed and give up the power. Suppose you just give God all of your anxiety and suffering and let Him do the carrying. And don't forget that God is in charge.

  Cognitive Renewal Statements: I give up on trying to manage the healing process. My future is in God's hands, and I am going to sleep soundly.

- ***Build an Aloha Ceremony to Relax and Sleep***
  Healing and tranquility are not possible in a madhouse. Trauma is a dust on our hearts, but it's also a dust on our bodies. To get a good, calm sleep, we need to make the space peaceful and comfortable.

  Your bedroom needs to function as your Zen space with your bed serving as your sanctuary. The purpose goes beyond physical health to create a relaxing atmosphere for both your body and mind. To relax fully, use calming scents with dimmed lighting and soothing soundtracks. As you prepare to sleep at night, declare to yourself that God's peace surrounds you and you remain protected under His care.

  Mindful Rest Practices: Make your bedroom a Zen Zone. Shut the lights off, sniff calming fragrances, and be sure your bed is a safe, secure spot where you can lie down.

  Cognitive Renewal Statements: I create a peaceful space for my body and mind to heal. I am safe in God's presence, and I rest knowing He is with me.

- ***Replace Negative Thoughts with God's Reality***
  When trauma has taken place, thoughts of the negative, anxious, and frightening kind can overwhelm the brain. Those thoughts are usually worse at night, so we can't sleep. But the truth of God is greater than all falsehood or fear.

31 Days to Overcoming Insomnia

We are told in Psalm 147:3 that God mends our wounds and Jeremiah 29:11 that God plans a good plan for us with hope and peace. Even when the suffering is terrible, we can choose to counter it with the reality of God's truth, which tells us that He loves, safeguards, and will work through us.

Mindful Rest Practices: When thoughts about being unwell creep in during the night, counteract them with Scripture or affirmations of God's truth. Let it be the voice in your head of the peace and hope God has for you.

Cognitive Renewal Statements: I cast out fear, and I replace it with the truth of God. He is healing my heart and His plans for me are so hopeful and peaceful.

- ***Breathe in the Strength of God's Healing Presence***
  That's the last step: be in the healing arms of God. Trauma takes time to recover, but God's calm and restoring grace works while you sleep. The promises of Psalm 147:3 are that God doesn't only heal partially, but He heals whole. He is repairing your heart, your brain, and your sleep. You can let yourself know that God is at work even if you don't believe it. Believe that every night you are on the road to completeness and serenity.

  Mindful Rest Practices: Before you go to bed, picture God's healing presence in your life, remaking you and making you still. Let go of the anxieties of the day and lie down in Him.

  Cognitive Renewal Statements: I sleep in God's healing breath. He has my heart in His hands, and I know He's healing my mind, body, and spirit.

Moving Toward Peaceful Sleep
When we're sleep-deprived from trauma, it's a process—a process of recovery, surrender, and faith. We have both Psalm 147:3 and Jeremiah 29:11 to remind us that God has a hand in healing us. He is doing His work of redeeming our souls, and His will for us is promising and tranquil.

You are from suffering to bliss— one step at a time, night after night. Because you will give God the pain and leave the tyranny in His hand, He will heal and quiet your soul. This is not a walk in the park to a good night's sleep, but it is a path that leads to wholeness, joy, and a future of God's ultimate tranquility.

Unlock Deep Sleep Secrets

Prayer for the Journey

Dear God, before I request Your assistance in the pursuit of sweet sleep tonight, I would like to say thank you for how You have been answering my prayers for sweet sleep. I can see Your power working in me to ensure that I get proper rest. I am so grateful. Now, tonight, I come before You hanging unto the promise You made in Psalms 47:3, that You have power to heal the brokenhearted like me and bind up my wounds.

Paps, no one knows me like You. You are the only one who sees my insecurities, hurts, cares, and anxiety that weigh me down. I rely on Your might to rebuild what is broken in my life and bring order to the chaos that causing sleeplessness in my life.

Lord, I ask you to personally and carefully tend to my heart and hurts. Please bring peace, restoration, and comfort to me just as a physician wraps a wound to promote healing. I know my sleepless nights somehow stem from being emotionally injured - unresolved issues, grief and anxiety- but I know that if You are powerful enough to rule the heavens then You can heal my wounded heart. Thank you for healing the wounds from my heart that cause me to struggle emotionally. You know the wounds I speak of and the silent ones I struggle to name. I surrender every sorrow and worry into Your hands. I bind the fear and anxious thoughts that keep me awake and replace them with Your peace the passes all understanding.

When I lay down tonight, blanket me with Your comforting presence. I speak peace to my mind, soothing to my spirit and restoration to my soul. I trust You to keep Your big eyes on me (LOL – I love you so much, Lord) as I sleep because You are truly my Protector and Healer...... In Jesus' name. Amen.

31 Days to Overcoming Insomnia

JOURNAL

"Sound Sleep is Important"

Morning Cognitive Renewal Statements

- I am on a journey from pain to peace, and I embrace the healing process.
- With God's help, I will find joy and hope in each day.
- I trust that healing is possible, and I am open to receiving it.

Morning Journal Guided Reflections

What is one step I can take today to nurture my emotional and physical well-being? How can I invite God into my healing journey today? What Does God's Word say about my trauma?

_____
_____
_____
_____
_____
_____
_____
_____
_____
_____
_____
_____
_____
_____
_____

Morning Mindful Rest Practices

Gratitude Journaling: Spend 5-10 minutes writing down three things you're grateful for, focusing on the positives in your life that contribute to healing.

- I am grateful for _____
- I am thankful for _____
- I appreciate for _____

Breath Awareness: Start your day with 5 minutes of deep breathing exercises, inhaling peace and exhaling tension.

Unlock Deep Sleep Secrets

Healthy Breakfast: Prepare a nourishing breakfast that fuels your body, such as oatmeal with fruits and nuts, to promote physical well-being.

Write: Jeremiah 29:11 and Psalm 137:4 on an index card and place it on your bathroom mirror. Say this scripture loud.

Evening vs Cognitive Renewal Statements

- I release the burdens of today and invite peace into my heart.
- I am grateful for the steps I took toward healing today.
- God's plans for me are filled with hope and a bright future.

Evening Guided Reflections

What moments of peace did I experience today despite my pain? How did I honor my feelings today, and what did I learn about my healing journey?

_____
_____
_____
_____
_____
_____
_____
_____
_____
_____
_____
_____
_____
_____
_____

Evening Mindful Rest Practices

- **Guided Meditation:** Spend 10-15 minutes in a guided meditation focused on healing and peace. You can find resources online or use an app for this.
- **Reflective Reading:** Read a chapter from a book or a few devotional entries that speak to healing and peace, allowing these words to sink in before bed.
- **Gentle Stretching:** Engage in 10 minutes of gentle stretching or yoga to release any physical tension accumulated throughout the day.
- **Scripture:** Repeat Jeremiah 29:11 and Psalm 137:4 out loud and meditate on it.

Day 25
FORGIVE YOURSELF AND SLEEP

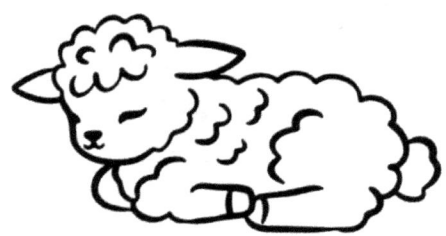

Matthew 11:28 (NIV):
"Come to me, all you who are weary and burdened, and I will give you rest."

The Hidden Weight of Guilt

Have you ever gone to sleep with your heart beating loud? That kind of heart, weighed down with guilt, or regret, or unaddressed self-recrimination? When your body gets into bed, you are in the middle of it, turning and spinning over the past, the wrongs you've done, and all the things you wish you could undo. It's like your flaws follow you to bed and you're up, jittery, unable to receive that rejuvenating rest you crave.

For guilt is one of the biggest rapists of good sleep. It hangs like a cloud over our heads and hearts and makes it difficult to calm down even if we're tired. But there is a solution, a way to break free of the guilt and wanderlust and forgive yourself. And the secret to that is Jesus' easy but powerful invitation at Matthew 11:28: "Come to me, you who work and are laden, and I will give you rest."

It promises to give you rest – physical, but also soul-rest – that one where guilt is released, spirit refilled, and you fall asleep. Tonight, you get to break that promise and release all the things preventing you from that amazing rest you so desire.

The Bondage of Unforgiveness

We all get it wrong, and sometimes those mistakes are very infected. Feeling guilty and sorry for decisions or actions that have infected you or others is normal. But the weight of that guilt in the backpack is like rock dust: it gets heavier by the day. The more time you carry it around, the less able you are to proceed, and the less peace you have when it is time to sleep.

Unlock Deep Sleep Secrets

That is where self-forgiveness steps in. Forgiveness is not resigning yourself or making it as if it never happened; forgiveness is deciding to give up the dominion your wrongs have over you. And if we are not forgiven, then the past festers inside us, and we can never truly inhabit the present—and therefore sleep at night.

It's just the reality of things. You can't undo the past, but you can decide to stop letting it define you. Forgiveness is something Jesus freely gives—and He will forgive you, too. Jesus says in Matthew 11:28 to put down all that weighs on you, especially that guilt you feel over your own transgressions, and let Him take it away from you.

The Healing Force of Forgiveness and Discipline

Forgiving yourself isn't a mental game, it's a spiritual one. To forgive means believing that God's mercy exceeds your own fall. You are acknowledging that God's love is free, and He wants you to be free—not stuck in shame or guilt.

Forgive yourself and you're able to move towards harmony. It is a peace not because of your goodness, but because of the love and forgiveness of God. His pardon isn't tied up in strings. It's given, and it's given fully and unconditionally; you just have to take it.

You not only forgive yourself, but you also rest. You let go of the emotional baggage that keeps your head fluttering and your heart racing so you can relax and sleep. The Bible says that peace comes after forgiveness. And when you forgive yourself, peace will be your friend, as you slide into the restorative sleep you seek.

From Shame to Freedom: Forgive and Calm the Self and Get Some Sleep!

Forgiving yourself can be tough if you've carried the guilt around your neck for a long time. But the good news is that God's forgiveness is immediate, and He desires you to feel the rest that comes with having been forgiven completely. How do you get started in forgiveness and sleeping tonight?

Here are some actionable steps for you to forgive yourself and get a good night's rest:

- *Acknowledge Your Guilt Without Shame*
  Start by naming the mistake or regret that you've been holding on to. Bring it before God unhated; let yourself feel the guilt, but do not be ruled by it. God knows you well, and He will forgive you. Don't forget that recognizing your guilt is not the same as allowing it to define you; it's just the first step to recovery.

  <u>Mindful Rest Practices:</u> As you sit in silence before God, write down what you are doing or thinking that is making you feel sleepy. Write them down, consider how

they've impacted you, and pray over them with God.

Cognitive Renewal Statements: I know I will make mistakes, but I won't be defined by them. I decide to let go of the guilt and be forgiven by God.

- **Surrender the Guilt to God**
  Once you've acknowledged your guilt, **surrender it to God.** Jesus offers rest, and that rest begins when you release what you cannot change. Trust that God has already forgiven you, and now it's time to let go of the burden of guilt. Trust that He is working in your life to bring healing and restoration.

  Mindful Rest Practices: Take a few moments to breathe deeply and imagine yourself laying down your guilt before God. Visualize releasing it from your heart and letting it go, trusting that He will handle it.

  Cognitive Renewal Statements: I surrender my guilt to God. I trust that He has forgiven me, and I choose to rest in His peace.

- **Embrace the Freedom of Forgiveness**
  Forgiveness is freedom. Forgive yourself and live in God's grace-freedom. Do not dwell on past errors because God doesn't blame you for them. To be liberated by God's forgiveness and to have it make you feel calm as you settle down for sleep.

  Mindful Rest Practices: Before going to bed, repeat to yourself *"I am forgiven, I am loved, and I am free."*

  Cognitive Renewal Statements: I embrace God's forgiveness. I am no longer guilt-ridden and I can go to bed at night.

- **Create a Calming Nighttime Ritual**
  Before going to sleep, create a peaceful space to help you forgive and rest. De-interrupt, dim lights, and set the intention to surrender the weight of the day. Think about adding a prayer, journal, or relaxation practice such as deep breathing to settle your thoughts and body.

  Mindful Rest Practices: Pray for a few minutes asking God for forgiveness and His peace as you sleep. Let go of any remaining feelings of regret or anxiety.

  Cognitive Renewal Statements: I go to sleep in the Lord tonight. I believe in His love, and I go to bed free of guilt.

Unlock Deep Sleep Secrets

Resting in Grace

Matt. 11:28 asks that you lay down your weight—especially guilt and self-denial. Jesus is giving you rest and rest is when you forgive yourself and believe in God's mercy. Forgiveness is a decision to allow your heart and soul to be at peace, and at peace, it is time to sleep well again.

This night when you lie down to sleep, know that you are forgiven. You do not have to be burdened by the sandbag of your shortcomings anymore. Give your all to God's love, let go of the guilt, and let the sacrament of forgiveness carry you into a good night's rest.

<u>Cognitive Renewal Statements:</u> I am forgiven, and I choose to rest in God's peace tonight. I release guilt and embrace His love. My sleep is a gift of grace.
Forgive yourself and sleep—peacefully, deeply, and restfully.

Prayer for the Journey

Dear God, it's me again coming to You this evening with much gratitude in my heart. Thank you for the compassionate invitation You extend to me in Matthew 11:28: "Come on to me you said, all who labor and are heavy burden and I will give you rest."

"Come unto me"

Lord, I'm coming to you tonight. I know You alone have the answer for sweet sleep. I have tried so many things to try to sleep. I have taken a lot of medication in an attempt to get good rest. Some worked partially; most of the others did not. I am here responding to Your personal appeal because You are the source of everything, even the source of good rest. I recognize that You are the Lord who gives me deep-rooted, sweet sleep.

"All ye that labour and are heavy laden"

Yes, Lord, I have been toiling and striving because of the burdens placed on me by life's challenges, namely stress, guilt, grief, or worry. I know my insomnia is due to the weight of unrelenting thoughts that I entertain – thoughts that come from regrets from the past, the pressures of daily life, and anxieties about my future.

"I will give you rest"

But I know You hold the remedy for good rest. Flood my soul with peace that surpasses understanding. Psalms 124:8 says our help is in the name of the Lord Jesus. So, I command my recent mind to be quiet in the name of Jesus, my heart to be calm in the name of Jesus, and Your soothing presence will woo me to perfect rest tonight in the name of Jesus.
Lord, as I lay tonight, let Your mercy surround me. I pray Your comfort will lead me to restful sleep. Restore my mind and body for the new day ahead, and I decree that I will awake refreshed, knowing that Your grace is sufficient, and Your love never fails. Amen and amen.

31 Days to Overcoming Insomnia

JOURNAL
"Sound Sleep is Important"

As you wake, recognize that self-forgiveness is an ongoing journey. Each morning offers a fresh start. Embrace the new day with a sense of lightness, knowing that you have released yesterday's burdens. This mindset fosters positivity and resilience, allowing you to move forward with confidence.

Morning Cognitive Renewal Statements

- I am worthy of love and forgiveness. Today, I embrace new possibilities with an open heart.

Morning Journal Guided Reflections

Take a moment to breathe deeply and set your intentions for the day. Reflect on the forgiveness you offered yourself the night before. How will you carry this into your actions today? Write down one positive affirmation that empowers you.

_____
_____
_____
_____
_____
_____
_____

Morning Mindful Rest Practices

Gratitude Practice: List three things you're grateful for to cultivate a positive mindset.

- I am grateful for _____
- I am thankful for _____
- I appreciate for _____

Stretching: Engage in gentle stretches to awaken your body and mind.

Mindful Breathing: Spend a few minutes focusing on your breathing to ground yourself for the day ahead.

Unlock Deep Sleep Secrets

Evening Cognitive Renewal Statements

- I forgive myself for my mistakes, understanding they do not define me. I am free to rest and recharge.

Evening Reflection
As the day ends, it's essential to create a space for self-forgiveness. Holding onto guilt or regret can weigh heavily on our minds, making it difficult to relax and drift into sleep. This time of reflection allows you to acknowledge your imperfections and understand that they are part of your growth. Forgiving yourself opens the door to peace, enabling a restful night.

Evening Journal Guided Reflections
Sit in a quiet space. Close your eyes and take a few deep breaths. Reflect on your day. Identify one thing you wish to forgive yourself for. Write down this acknowledgment and how it made you feel. Conclude with a note of gratitude for the lessons learned.

_____
_____
_____
_____
_____
_____
_____
_____

Evening Mindful Rest Practices

Letter of Forgiveness: Write a letter to yourself expressing forgiveness.

_____
_____
_____
_____
_____
_____
_____
_____

Meditation: Spend 5-10 minutes in guided meditation focused on letting go of burdens.

Day 26
THE WORD IN ACTION: BRINGING SCRIPTURE TO LIFE

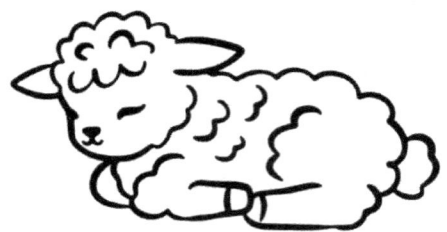

2 Timothy 2:15 (NKJV):
*"Be diligent to present yourself approved to God,
a worker who does not need to be ashamed,
rightly dividing the word of truth."*

When the world is crashing into your head and sleep is an unaffordable comfort, God's Word can set you at ease, soothe you, and give you rest. Sleep is a lost cause when we're too busy, a second that goes by in the blink of an eye when we're up, thinking and thinking. What if, however, I was to reveal to you that the secret to good, restful sleep is not in a pillow or a nighttime routine, but in the Scriptures that you hold in your hands? And what if God's Word put to work, can still your heart, soothe your body, and give you the deep sleep you've been waiting for?

God's Word Is a Force to Be Struck With: More Than Words
Paul tells us, in 2 Timothy 2:15, to be diligent, that we might come before God holiness, according as the Word of truth is divided rightly. This is not intellectual knowing, but it is using the Word thoughtfully and intentionally. "Rightly dividing" is to interpret and live the Word of God according to the letter of the Scripture in every way possible. And that goes for your sleep, too.

If we read the Scriptures closely, then we're not just being taught life lessons; we're being taught to make it through the tribulations of life with wisdom, power, and peace. And when we need to battle for rest, God's Word is our best friend. We have to work hard to read the Bible, and we should work hard to put it into practice when we try to get some good sleep.

Scripture As a Way of Rest
Peace is the greatest good in the present. We can be so deprived of sleep by anxiety, stress,

Unlock Deep Sleep Secrets

and performing, or just constantly being tossed awake in an undisciplined way. And this is the wonderful thing: the Word of God can make a difference that no words can explain.

Philippians 4:6-7 states, *"Do not be anxious about anything, but in all by prayer and supplication, with thanksgiving let your requests be known to God; and the peace of God which passes all understanding will guard your hearts and minds through Christ Jesus."*

And that is not just for prayer in the daytime—it is also for night time, when your thoughts run and your heart can hardly stand still. You rightly divide the Word of truth, and you come to realize that peace is with you night after night. When you utter God's Word over your life, you are requesting His peace to guard your heart and your mind and allow you to sleep in Him.

Rightly Cutting the Word for Sleep

So how do you split the Word of truth for good sleep? It starts with intentional application. There are promises and prayers in Scripture that are directly addressed to our need for rest, safety, and renewal. The Scriptures are not to be read, but lived out, and embraced, as you invite God into your world and hope that He can be the one who can rest your suffering soul.

One of the best Scriptures for sleep is Psalm 4:8: *"I will both lie down in peace, and sleep; For You alone, O Lord, make me dwell in safety."* This is a proclamation, a fact that you get to hold over your life every night. When you read out this verse, you are listening to the Word of God as you remind yourself that peace and safety are yours from the Creator of the world. Your sleep is not only a physiological rest, but it's also a spiritual surrender, where you believe God is in charge of all your things including your sleep.

So, also Psalm 127:2 should be your best friend when you can't sleep: *"It is vain for you to rise up early, to sit up late, to eat the bread of sorrows; for so He gives His beloved sleep."* God is good, and so He gives His beloved sleep. And it isn't something we need to deserve; it is something we need to be given. This Scripture is for those times of stress or restlessness, and it is a soft plea to let God's provision suffice you and ask Him to give you the night you need to be revivified.

Practical Advice on How to Get Proper Sleep from the Bible

How do we put the Word of God to work so that we're getting to sleep peacefully? It's not just knowing the song, but it's actually making it part of our nightly rhythm. Let's take a closer look at some practical things you can do to use Scripture to get real and have the rest you've been missing:

Meditate on God's Promises
Before closing your eyes, ponder for a few minutes on God's promises concerning sleep and calm, such as Psalm 4:8, Philippians 4:6-7, and Isaiah 26:3 – *"Ye will keep*

31 Days to Overcoming Insomnia

him in perfect peace, whose mind is stayed on You, because he trusts in You." Meditate on those verses, and the anxiety will be replaced by God's peace.

Declare His Rest Over Your Mind
You can say this as you're lying in bed, *"The tranquility of God is on my heart and my mind. And I will sleep soundly because of You, O Lord, cause me to sleep soundly."* When you say these words, you are listening to the Word of God and making God rest in your sleep.

Release Your Worries to God
Stress kills our sleep because we are told that we have to fix everything. But as God instructs us in Matthew 11:28-29, "Seek ye therefore when ye are tired and heavy laden and he will rest you." Just lay down your troubles before bed at His feet. Be able to know that He is on your side during the night and let Him handle the loads that keep you awake.

Pray for Comfort and Rest
Pray during the nighttime for peace, rest, and reconciliation. Request that God refresh your mind and body when you go to sleep because God always puts His children to sleep. Believe that when you go to sleep, He is at work restoring your strength for the day.

Create a Restful Environment
Words are good, but so is making the bed. Remove the screens, dim the lights, and create a calm bedroom. And when you are setting up, don't lose sight of the fact that you are not just setting up your physical space, but you are also letting God enter into the room and bless it with His presence.

The Word of God in Practice: Good Sleep is a Gift from God

God's Word is more than a living guide; it's a means of rest in every area of our lives including our sleep. If we do rightly divide the Word, we receive His words and apply them to our nights' rest. The Bible is filled with life-giving truths to quiet our fretful minds and our troubled hearts and get us back to serenity.

As you put the Word of God on your pillow, don't forget that sleep is not an extravagance or an afterthought; it is a gift. God made us to sleep and when we apply the Word to our lives, we can have the kind of deep, restful sleep He desires for us. Every time you sing it, every time you pray, every time you surrender, you are bringing God's quiet into your heart. So, the next time you are awake, trying to fall asleep, take heart that God's Word is not dead. It can give peace that's beyond understanding, and once you put it into practice, it will make your nights into a restful, healing time with the Lord.

Unlock Deep Sleep Secrets

Sleep is not physical rest; it's sleeping on His promises. And then you will sleep the kind of sleep where you wake up feeling clean and refreshed for the new day because you know God is with you at every hour, even in the dark of the night.

Prayer for the Journey

Dear God, as this day comes to an end and before I lay my head on this pillow, I am reminded that Your word is my firm foundation. I know that You are in complete control and Your promises are yes and amen. True peace comes when my heart and mind are aligned with Your word. The anxiety and restlessness that I experience stem from a sense of spiritual disconnection, leading to fear and confusion. However, at this moment, tonight, I submit myself to Your guidance, seeking solace in Your word. I decree that my mind is quiet from the noise of the day and I'm filled with the assurance that I am safe in Your arms.

Help me learn to study so I will be able to rightly divide Your word in order to anchor myself in Your promises. When I know Your word, I'll be able to silence the lies that caused me to toss and turn at night. Lord, in the same way You instructed Timothy through the apostle Paul, help me to diligently study Your word and live a life approved by You. Let Your truth anchor my heart so that every fear, worry, and doubt that try to steal my sleep will be cast out.

Tonight, I decree that I will have sound sleep without interruption because Your word is alive on the inside of me. I believe it is working powerfully to transform my heart. my mind, and my actions, and every promise in the scriptures is active in my life as I meditate on Your word in Jesús' name. Amen.

31 Days to Overcoming Insomnia

JOURNAL
"Sound Sleep is Important"

By engaging with the idea that "The Word of God will not return void," you cultivate a sense of peace and assurance in your life. This practice not only prepares your mind for restful sleep, but it also strengthens your faith, grounding you in the transformative power of God's promises.

Morning Cognitive Renewal Statements

- Today, I trust in the power of God's Word. It is alive and active in my life, bringing purpose and fulfillment.

Morning Journal Guided Reflections

Reflection: Take a moment to meditate on the meaning of God's promises. What does it mean to you that His Word does not return void? Consider the areas of your life where you seek His guidance and trust in His promise.

Morning Mindful Rest Practices

- **Quiet Time:** Spend 10-15 minutes in prayer, asking God to reveal areas where His Word can bring transformation in your life.
- **Scripture Reading:** Read Isaiah 55 and other passages that speak to the reliability of God's promises (e.g., Psalm 119:105, Matthew 24:35).
- **Gratitude Journaling:** Write down three things you are grateful for, focusing on how God's Word has impacted your life.

    - I am grateful for _____
    - I am thankful for _____
    - I appreciate for _____

Afternoon Mindful Rest Practices

Nature Walk: Take a walk outdoors and reflect on the beauty of creation as a testament to God's faithfulness. Allow the peace of the moment to wash over you, grounding you in the assurance of His promises.

Unlock Deep Sleep Secrets

Evening Cognitive Renewal Statements

- As I rest tonight, I trust that God's Word is at work in me, shaping my life and fulfilling His good purpose.

Evening Journal Guided Reflections

Reflection: As you wind down, think about the ways you saw God's Word at work today. Did you notice any moments where His promises were fulfilled? How did you experience His presence?

_____
_____
_____
_____
_____

Evening Mindful Rest Practices

- **Meditation:** Spend a few minutes in silence, reflecting on the day. Consider how God's Word has been a guide and a source of strength for you.
- **Prayer:** Close your day in prayer, asking God to help you trust in His word more deeply and to remind you of His promises as you sleep.
- **Sleep Preparation:** Create a calming bedtime routine—dim the lights, turn off screens, and perhaps read a comforting passage of Scripture.

Day 27
NOT TODAY, DEVIL:
CLAIMING VICTORY OVER OUR SLEEP

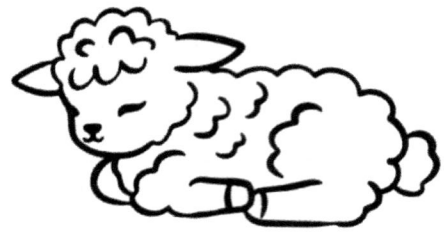

James 4:7 (NIV):
"Submit yourselves, then, to God. Resist the devil, and he will flee from you."

1 Peter 5:8-9 (NIV):
"Be alert and of sober mind. Your enemy the devil prowls around like a roaring lion looking for someone to devour. Resist him, standing firm in the faith, because you know that the family of believers throughout the world is undergoing the same kind of sufferings."

Among today's world of noise, terror, and anxiety, the pursuit of sound and restful sleep feels like an uphill battle. But what if I said you don't have to fall into sleep, you can own it? Wouldn't it be nice if, when you went to bed, you could say: "Not today, Devil!" because God has already won you over every alarm, every troubling thought, every adversary that wants to kill you?

And we as believers have the power to fight against the enemy every day—even during sleep. We can be strong in the Word of God and use it to proclaim victory over the enemy. The Battle for Your Sleep is an unlikely terrain, but the enemy knows how potent sleep can be. When you are rested, you are energized, renewed and ready for the challenge of the next day. He wants to kill you because if you're tired, he knows, you're ineffective, unresponsive, and prone to attacks.

But here's the good news: the devil can't stop you from sleeping if you don't allow him to. The Bible tells us that the enemy is like a roaring lion that is looking for someone to eat, but it also says that if you are repelled by him, he will leave you. When you are faithful in Christ and make Him your life's guarantor, then you don't have to suffer the nights. You can say,

Unlock Deep Sleep Secrets

"Not today, Devil!" and get your sleep back. And have a calm, sound sleep that the devil can't get away with.

Submit to God

James 4:7 is a powerful instruction: *"Submit to God. Stop the devil and he will run from you."* Humility to God is the best way to defeat the enemy's hoop. To submit is to bow down, know that we are in His protection and care, and live as He wills. When we do, God's peace fills our hearts and minds.

And so, as you go to bed, give your thoughts, fears, and worries to God. This is not just a prayer for sleep; it is to ask God to take charge of your whole night. With that realization that He's in charge, you close the door on whatever spiritual attacks the enemy tries to throw at you.

Resist the Devil: Have Power Over Your Sleep

We're told in 1 Peter 5:8-9 to "be drunk and wary" as the devil is always lurking, ready to strike. But the key here is the injunction to kill him. To 'do something against' the devil is to "do something against" any negative/destructive thoughts, fears, or distracting thoughts that would be trying to keep you from sleeping.

What do you do against the devil when you're asleep? That's easy, but powerful: speak the Word of God. When the devil is trying to agitate worry or fear in you, say loudly: "Not today, Devil!"

Attack from the Scriptures:

- **Psalm 4:8 (KJV)** – *"I will lay down in safety both, and sleep; For Only with You, Lord, do I live in safety."*
- **Isaiah 26:3 (KJV)** – *"You will keep him in peace, who minds have stayed to Thee, for he has put his confidence in Thee."*
- **Philippians 4:6-7 (KJV)** – *"Hurry not for nothing, but in everything through prayer and supplication, with thanksgiving, let your prayers be known to God; and the peace of God, which is above all knowledge, will guard your hearts and minds by Christ Jesus."*

These aren't pretty poems—they're spiritual bombs. When you utter them, you are fighting back against the enemy's attempts to disturb your tranquility. And you're saying you'll let God watch over your heart and your head and that only He can keep you through the night and protect your sleep.

31 Days to Overcoming Insomnia

Be Bold in Your Belief: You Will Win This Game

1 Peter 5:9 says to persevere in the faith because what is troubled in our lives is troubled in the world. This is critical: you're not the only one fighting. When the devil is trying to make you fearful, nervous, or uneasy, do not give up on your faith because God's peace is more effective than any demonic attack, he can throw at you.

Faith is your shield. As the Bible puts it: *"Faith is the substance of things hoped for, the evidence of things not seen"* (Hebrews 11:1). And by being unwavering in faith, you say you do not deny that God's promises are true, even when you can't quite see them. When it comes to bed, that means believing God will have your night, that He is doing work in the midst of your sleep, and that His quiet will be with you.

Prayer for the Journey

Dear God, as I lay down to sleep this evening, according to James 4:7, I totally submit myself to Your will and authority. I resist the devil's attempt to steal my peace. Lord, I realize spiritual battles don't end when I lie down at night. I am so tired of the worry, fear, and anxiety that creep in during the quiet hours to rob me of my sleep. So now that I am under submission, I decree that my heart is aligned with Your peace, and I reject every anxious thought, fear, or lie that contradicts the promises found in Your word. I know the security of God's presence now stands guard over my heart.

Jesus, I am aware that the devil lurks in the background like a roaring lion because he desires to steal my peace through worry, anxiety, and fear. I decree Satan has no authority over my mind, my rest, or my home. I stand firm in my faith in God and declare that I am covered in the blood of Jesus.

Every lie that tries to whisper fear into my heart, I resist. Every thought that contradicts Your promises, I reject. At this very moment, I embrace Your peace. Thank you for Your angels that encamp around me. Thank you for Your presence that shields me. Lord, I decree that my soul is quieted by Your presence. Please grant me sweet, undisturbed sleep in Jesus' name. Amen.

Unlock Deep Sleep Secrets

JOURNAL
"Sound Sleep is Important"

Morning Cognitive Renewal Statements

- Today, I submit to God and choose to resist negativity and fear. I declare, 'Not today, Devil!' I walk in faith and confidence, knowing that I am protected.

Morning Journal Guided Reflections

Reflect on Your Intentions: What are your intentions for today? Identify any potential challenges you may face and how you plan to resist them.

_____
_____
_____
_____

Identify Triggers: What thoughts or situations tend to lead you into negativity? Write them down and prepare to combat them with Scripture.

_____
_____
_____
_____

Evening Journal Guided Reflections

Evaluate Your Day: How did you resist the challenges you faced today? Reflect on specific moments where you declared "Not Today, Devil!" and stood firm in your faith.

_____
_____
_____
_____

Celebrate Victories: What victories, big or small, did you experience today? Acknowledge these moments as evidence of your strength.

_____
_____
_____
_____

31 Days to Overcoming Insomnia

Scriptures for Sleep: Fight with the Word

Have a set of verses by your bedside and meditate on them before sleep. They will be your spiritual weapons when the enemy tries to invade your thoughts.

- **Psalm 91:1-2** (KJV)– *"He who dwells in the secret place of the Most High shall abide under the shadow of the Almighty. I will say of the Lord, 'He is my refuge and my fortress; My God, in Him I will trust.'"*
- **Isaiah 41:10 (ESV)** – *"Fear not, for I am with you; Be not dismayed, for I am your God. I will strengthen you, Yes, I will help you, I will uphold you with My righteous right hand."*

Evening Cognitive Renewal Statements

- As I lay down to sleep, I release the struggles of the day. I have stood firm against the enemy, and I find peace in God's promises. Not today, Devil!

Evening Mindful Rest Practices

- **Mindfulness Meditation:** Spend a few minutes in quiet meditation. Focus on your breath and visualize pushing away negative thoughts, declaring *"Not today, Devil!"* with each exhale.
- **Scripture Reading:** Choose a quiet space and read James 4:7 and 1 Peter 5:8-9 aloud. Reflect on their meanings and how they apply to your life.
- **Journaling Exercise:** Write a short letter to the devil, expressing your determination to resist his influence in your life. Conclude with a statement of your commitment to God and your goals.

Unlock Deep Sleep Secrets

- **Physical Activity:** Engage in a short workout or yoga session. As you move, visualize any negativity or stress leaving your body, affirming your strength and resilience.
- **Gratitude List:** Before sleep, write down three things you are grateful for today. Focus on the positive aspects of your day to cultivate a peaceful mindset.

    - I am grateful for _____
    - I am thankful for _____
    - I appreciate for _____

Day 28
BEYOND THE 31 NIGHTS: A LASTING COMMITMENT TO REST

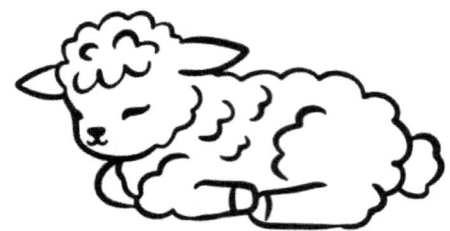

Galatians 6:4-5 (NIV):
"Each one should test their own actions. Then they can take pride in themselves alone, without comparing themselves to someone else, for each one should carry their own load."

The 31-night challenge might have been your launching pad, your first moment of action to take back your sleep, your silence, and your sleep. You may have known what it feels like to wake up with your head lighter, your mind sane and your body revitalized. But here's the deal: 31 nights doesn't mark the end of the road to uninterrupted sound sleep. And indeed, it's only the first part of a lifelong sleep-embrace.

All too often we resolve to do something now, but we lose sight of it when life gets busy or challenging. But only by crossing paths with indeterminate endeavors can we really change. Sound sleep is not a temporary dream— it's an investment in ourselves, our health, and our mental health.

We will learn how to make a commitment to rest that can be kept, with the eternal counsel of Scripture on our side. Here, we will read Galatians 6:4-5, teaching us personal accountability, work and introspection to achieve the life of rest. Let's figure out how to continue the habits of sleep we've worked so hard to build and cement them as a permanent part of our lives.

How to Own Your Sleep: Taking Ownership of Your Rest
In Galatians 6:4-5, Apostle Paul is asking us to review ourselves and own up to what we do: *"But let each one see his work, and then he will rejoice in himself alone, and not in another. For every one of us shall take up his own burden."* This Scripture doesn't just apply to what we do or do work for, but it also applies to how we treat our own health and well-being – including sleep. The scripture invites us to become personal stewards of our

Unlock Deep Sleep Secrets

own lives. You have no one else who can "carry your load" when it comes to sleep. You can get support or advice from other people, but you must decide to live by a sleeping-heaven's light.

That is the point of not staying on the 31 nights. You're choosing to stay the course, even when it's too much to digest, or life threatens to re-engineer you. We all revert to old habits, but if we look at our own "work" (and here, it is our work of getting more sleep), we'll see that the happiness and relaxation of a good night's sleep is worth the effort every night.

Reflecting on Where You've Been: Accountability Through the Obstacle
How to maintain your new sleep routine: It begins with regular assessments of your progress. Galatians 6:4 hints at self-examination: *"Let each one take a look at his work."* We must check our sleeping routine in the same way that we check our body in a workout program.

Ask yourself:

What have I been like since waking up?
Has it improved my energy, mood, or health?
What have I been able to do to sleep well consistently?
How do I change or tweak my habits so that the change sticks?

Reflection helps you to look in the mirror and look at your habits squarely and make changes. Not only does this action demonstrate you are on the right track, but it also reminds you why you came to this place in the first place— to live a life of peace, health, and aliveness.

Stopping the Drive to Fall Back into Old Habits
The temptation to revert will be there. There will be snags in your life— work, kids, the nights when you just can't go to sleep. But sleep commitment calls for relentless work and for you to not allow the devil to steal your sleep.

'For each one shall bear his own load,' says Galatians 6:5, for we can turn to others for advice and help, but it is up to us to provide for our rest. We should not give into temptation to return to old ways of keeping peace.

For that, don't lose track of how you sleep. Learn techniques for those hard nights. Maybe you're in need of some Zen meditation, like a prayer before bed or some breathing exercises. Or maybe you need to take a fresh look at your world—is there something in the way, and it isn't relaxing your body and brain? Protect sleep, draw boundaries, and do it every day without exception.

31 Days to Overcoming Insomnia

The more often you commit to these habits, the less of a tool the enemy has to break your peace.

Setting New Habits for Long-Term Sleep: Create New Habits for Sleep
Once you're out of the 31 nights, you have to get back into a sustainable habit. Consistency is the secret to successful loyalty. Healthy sleep habits aren't like starting a new exercise routine or eating well—they're taking time, work, and a schedule.

These are some ways you can develop a habit of sleep that will last:

Establish a regular bedtime and waking time: Like you'd put your workouts at the top of your agenda, make sure your sleep is, too. Getting to sleep and waking up in the same time every day also keep your body on track.

You should sleep well: Your bedroom is the place to sleep. Cool, dark, and silent. Avoid screen time before bed and take away anything that can get in the way of your sleep.

Work in sleep-inducing activities: Do some calming activities before bed like reading scripture, listening to soothing music, or writing down thoughts. This is your body telling you to relax.

Stay hydrated: Your body health is the biggest influence on how well you sleep. Take care of yourself with daily exercise, healthy eating, and managed stress levels to keep yourself in the sort of condition that ensures you fall asleep.

The Reward of Lasting Rest
The price you pay for your commitment isn't a decent night's sleep, but the ability to live life to the fullest. A good night's sleep influences everything: your mood, your productivity, your friends and family, even your health. When you sleep first, God can restore you.

Psalm 4:8 says: I will both sleep with ye, and be a sound sleep; For You alone, O Lord, set me to sleep in safety. When you commit to sleeping for a lifetime, you are contributing to God's plan for you. Sleep is a time of worship in which He re-energizes and heals you so that you can face the day with difficulty and pleasure.

Embracing the Journey of Rest
The path to enduring rest is not a sprint— it's a marathon. It takes hard work, reflection, and total trust in God as with any other endeavor to make progress in life. That 31-night challenge was the start, but the magic is in the fact that sleep becomes a part of your life for good, that you decide no matter what, you will secure your peace and rest.

Unlock Deep Sleep Secrets

Once you get past the 31 nights, use Galatians 6:4-5 to help you: "Always check yourself", and "bear your own burden." Own your sleep knowing that each night you spend in restful sleep is a day towards greater health, happiness, and power.

Make today your bedtime promise, one that will see you out of this hole into one of peace, vitality, and vibrancy. Sleep well, knowing that your body, mind, and soul are being refilled, reformed, and remade each and every night.

Prayer for the Journey

Dear God, thank you for the precious reminder You give me in Galatians 6:4-5. I did not realize that I needed to prove my own work, that is, I needed to examine my own actions to ensure that they aligned with Your will. I now understand that if I fail to do so, then I might compare myself to others. Instead of focusing on my own faithfulness to You, Lord, I ask for Your forgiveness. Whether my struggle to rest at night is because my mind is weighed down with comparisons, worries, or pressures to perform, please show me. In this world, it is so easy to measure our worth against others, whether through social status or financial success, or even spiritual growth. Now I understand this important truth, that You called me to focus on my own walk with You rather than measuring myself by someone else's progress.

As of now, I trust that my faithfulness is what matters to You. I choose to faithfully focus on doing what You have placed before me rather than striving to meet the expectations of others, because in doing so, I will find the peace I need for a restful evening, the peace that leads to sweet sleep. I now decree that I'm free from the weight of comparison, the weight of self-doubt, and the weight of unnecessary burdens.

As I close my eyes this evening, I release every unnecessary burden and embrace the peace of God. I am called to walk my own journey with the Lord, so I do not compare myself with others. Now that I know God is pleased with my faithfulness, I'm going to sleep peacefully in Jesus' name. Amen.

31 Days to Overcoming Insomnia

JOURNAL
"Sound Sleep is Important"

Cognitive Renewal Statements

- I am accountable for my sleep and I will always improve in sleeping well. And I'm closer to the sleep that cleanses my body, my mind, and my soul every night.

Guided Reflections
Take 10 minutes tonight before going to bed to ask yourself the following questions:

Reflecting on Your Progress: Accountability Beyond the Challenge

- What did I feel when I woke up these last couple of nights?
- Are my energy, mood, or health feeling better?
- So, how have I stayed consistent with rest?
- How do I change or modify my habit to make lasting changes?
- Write in a sleep diary to record what you think and feel. Your own review of the process is important so that you are on board and have a toolbox for when you need to adjust.

Resisting the Urge to Slip Back into Old Patterns

Activity to Build Strength: The 5-Minute Wind-Down Workout
Whenever you want to go back to what you've been doing or your mind starts to race at night, try this 5-minute wind-down sequence:

- ***Turn off everything electronic:*** Unplug all the things that interfere with your serenity.
- ***Let's just sit for a moment and inhale:*** Take 4 deep breaths in through your nose, rest 4 for 4, and then slowly out of your mouth 6 times.
- ***Restore sanity:*** Say this mantra as you exhale—"The peace of God keeps my heart and mind. I will rest tonight."
- ***Text of comfort:*** Pick your go-to Scripture for rest, a favorite being Psalm 4:8 —"I will both sleep in peace, and fall asleep; For You alone, O Lord, make me dwell in safety. It clears your mind and gets your body ready for sleep.

Unlock Deep Sleep Secrets

Cognitive Renewal Statements for Resistance

- I fight everything distraction and bad thought. I have slept instead of worried and give my rest to God.

Establishing New Routines for Long-Term Rest

Here are a few tips to make a lasting sleeping routine:

- ***Set a regular bedtime and wake-up time:*** Getting to bed and getting up in the same time each day keeps your body in the proper rhythm.
- ***Build a quiet bedroom:*** Make your bedroom a sleeping space. Keep it cool, dark, and silent. Do not watch screens before bed and don't engage in any other activity that could disturb your sleeping.
- ***Add sleep-enhancing activities:*** Before bed, do things to relax like reading Scripture, listening to soft music, or writing down your thoughts. This tells your body it's time to settle down.
- ***Stay in good shape:*** You have to keep your body healthy to get the best sleep possible. You need to run, eat right, and control your stress to be in the kind of health that makes you go to sleep.

Prompt for Routine Building
What are 3 sleep-supporting habits that you can work towards next month? They're written down and you can make sure to remind yourself of them so you can work them into your day.

Affirmation for Routine
I make a pledge to get a good night's sleep. Every night, I set the stage and make peace a priority, my body and mind both need that time to reset.

Final Thought
There is no room for sleep; it is imperative. Take that step to sleep with intention and purpose, and you'll go a long way. Your serenity is well worth the trouble, and in God's name, your sleep will never be broken, day after day, night after night.

Day 29
RESTORING PEACE: LETTING GO OF GRUDGES BEFORE BED

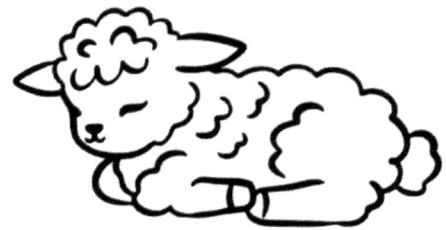

Ephesians 4:31 (NIV):
"Get rid of all bitterness, rage and anger, brawling and slander, along with every form of malice."

Sleep is one of the deepest recharges our brains and bodies have. Yet sometimes we go to bed bursting with anger or bitterness—emotions that sabotage our tranquility and eviscerate the sleep we so desperately crave. You might carry angry words or disappointments or unresolved conflicts around with you all day long, but when they are stuck in our hearts as we fall asleep, they eat at us while ruining our sleep and well-being.

Paul tells us in Ephesians 4:31 to "get rid of" bad feelings such as anger, resentment, anger, clamour, and vitriol. This Scripture has no doubt to do with how we can make ourselves and relationships peaceful again. The thing is, if we have any resentments, if we have any negative feelings, it's only going to make us go to sleep rolling over with things we can't resolve. But when we release those negative feelings, we free up the space to allow for good sleep.

This workbook will explain why you should forget things before bed so that you can sleep better, get up again, and be a good soul. So, let's see how Ephesians 4:31 can help us let go of the rotten feelings that stand in our way of sleep so that healing and peace can ensue.

The Cost of Resentments: What They Do to Your Sleep

Grudges do not just take up room in your head—they take up space in your heart. Instinct and resentment are heavy weights to be burdened by. It's exhausting, mentally and physically. And, alas, that feeling doesn't vaporize just because the sun sets. They can track you through the night, occupying your rest and making you sleepless.

Unlock Deep Sleep Secrets

We can read Ephesians 4:31 right here about this: *"Let all bitterness, wrath, anger, clamor, and evil speaking be put away from you."* Here, "bitterness" means a cruel, bitter nature. If we let anger rot, it's toxic—not just to our relationships, but to our sleep. Stoking anger and resentment is only making the emotion stronger, which makes it more repressive in our heart.

Leaving Behind Resentment: Making a Choice to Go Away with Peace
Grudges don't always come easy. To be forgiven is a struggle when one feels cheated, and it seems as if we're relinquishing something when we release our anger. But the reality is, that resentment does us no good. It keeps us trapped in the negativity cycle and robs us of the joy God intends for us.

Ephesians 4:31 is not a proposal but a command. God doesn't want us carrying around emotional weight that makes it hard to sleep or be in relationships. Rather, He invites us to lay them aside, so we may live in freedom—without anger, spite, and hatred. Forgiveness and letting go are decisions we have to make, not on our own merits, but on God's.

God's Promise of Peaceful Rest
That is the peace that disarming of anger offers, a God-given peace, a peace that surpasses comprehension and hearts. *'And the peace of God, which surpasses all understanding,'* writes Paul in Philippians 4:7, *'will guard your hearts and minds through Christ Jesus.'* If we forgive and let go of resentment, we will be subject to the peace of God, who will guard our hearts and minds so that we can sleep peacefully.

And Psalm 4:8 adds to this: *"I will both sleep in safety, and lay down; For You alone, O Lord, give me rest in safety."* God has the peace and safety of His presence, and when we put aside the burdens of our revenges, we're putting ourselves into this kind of rest.

When we remove the resentment baggage of unforgiveness, we allow God's peace to surround us. It is not our hearts and minds that are slaves to anger, bitterness, and resentment. This quiet is not an outcome of our circumstances; it's the grace of God to sleep with him.

The Transformative Power of Forgiveness
Forgiveness doesn't just save relationships; it saves us. And when we do release grudges, we have the choice of feeling the release that heals the soul. Forgiveness can be a healing balm, not only with others, but with us. It softens our hearts, eases our stress, and gives us sleep.

Repressed anger and resentment don't change history—it makes us stuck. But in

31 Days to Overcoming Insomnia

forgiveness, we exit the cycle of negativity and free ourselves to experience the present in harmony and happiness.

Embracing Restful, Grudge-Free Sleep
While you are about to sleep tonight, say that you have made the choice to be a grudge-free person. Give up all that is bitter and angry and let God's love rest on your heart. As we are reminded in Matthew 11:28: *"Come to Me, all you who labor and are heavy laden, and I will give you rest."* By abandoning the emotional world, we are left with the rest only Christ can give. Our hearts are less heavy, our minds less clouded, and we sleep calmer and more rejuvenated.

Prayer for the Journey
Dear God, tonight, I will make room for Your peace to fill my heart and my mind. Tonight, I choose to let go for restful sleep. No longer will I lay awake at night replaying a conversation, reliving a hurt, or feeling the weight of unresolved emotions. Lord. You know sometimes my mind refuses to shut down because it's trapped in a cycle of frustration and unrest. Lord, I realize the truth is, bitterness, anger, and unforgiveness are burdens too heavy for me to carry, and it has robbed me of the rest You desire for me. Tonight, I am letting go. In Ephesians 4:31, You command us to put away all bitterness, wrath, anger, clamor, and evil speaking with all malice — I am putting these emotions away tonight. I choose to forgive NOW. No more resentment. It stops now; I surrender.

I trust Your justice and release these toxic emotions that steal my inner peace. Holy Spirit, I ask You to empower me to cleanse my heart of these negative emotions so that I can experience divine rest and peace. I can't do this on my own. I need Your help so I can experience the rest of God. Now, I decree my heart feels light and my mind remains calm as my spirit experiences renewal this night. Because I have released the day's offenses, my sleep will now be sweet and restorative.

I thank you, Lord, because You show me how to forgive others and extend mercy. Every injury I carry is surrendered to You so that You may provide healing and restoration. Tonight, I lie down in Your perfect peace with eyes closed and wake up tomorrow with abundant love and gratitude in my heart. I pray and decree this truth in Jesus' powerful name. Amen.

Unlock Deep Sleep Secrets

JOURNAL
"Sound Sleep is Important"

Morning Journal Guided Reflections

Identifying Resentments

So, take a moment now and reflect on any leftover quarrels, enmities, or hurts you might have. Ask yourself: So, who/what is making me resentful? How does this resentment make me sleep or feel restless? How might we release this trauma tonight? Writing out your thoughts can tell you where your emotional weight comes from and what needs to go into the closet.

_____
_____
_____
_____
_____
_____
_____
_____
_____
_____
_____
_____
_____
_____
_____

Cognitive Renewal Statements of Release

Create a morning affirmation inspired by Ephesians 4:31, such as: *"Today, I choose to release all bitterness and anger, allowing peace to fill my heart."*

_____
_____
_____
_____

Intentions for the Day

Set an intention to approach any challenging interactions today with grace and forgiveness. How can you practice kindness, even when it's difficult?

_____
_____
_____
_____

31 Days to Overcoming Insomnia

Gratitude Focus

List three things you are grateful for this morning.
- I am grateful for _____
- I am thankful for _____
- I appreciate for _____

How do these blessings help shift your perspective away from resentment?
_____
_____
_____
_____
_____
_____

Afternoon Journal Guided Reflections

Midday Reflection
Take a moment to assess your day. Have you encountered situations that reignited feelings of resentment? _____ Write about how you responded.
_____
_____
_____
_____
_____
_____

Releasing Negative Emotions
Identify a specific instance where you felt anger or bitterness today. Write a brief letter to the person or situation expressing your feelings, then set it aside as a symbolic gesture of release.

Prayer for Forgiveness
Write a prayer asking God to help you let go of resentment and fill your heart with peace. Be specific about the emotions you want to release.
_____
_____
_____
_____
_____
_____

Unlock Deep Sleep Secrets

Encouragement
Reach out to a friend or family member and share your journey of letting go of resentment. Offer encouragement to each other in pursuing peace.

Evening Mindful Rest Practices

- **Exercise: The "Stand Back and Let Go" Ritual:** This is the quick, easy way to wash your heart of all anger and grudges tonight, before going to bed:
    - Sit in a place that is peaceful and peaceful.
    - Just close your eyes and breathe deep to calm the brain and body.
    - Think of the person or circumstance that made you unhappy or bitter. Recognize the injury, but rather than carry it around, imagine releasing it.
    - Repeat: With your mouth or in your heart: *"I am letting go of this anger and resentment Father. I forgive [name or situation]. 'I turn over this wound to You because You're in charge. I put my heart in You and my quiet."*
    - Go in again and on the exhale, picture the resentment draining out of your body, replaced by quiet.
    - Declare: *"I choose peace tonight, and I will sleep in the freedom of forgiveness."* Repeat.
    - The mere act of declaring it will move you from the angry state into the tranquil state of rest in the arms of God.
- **Meditative Journaling:** Spend time journaling about your feelings of resentment. Allow yourself to express everything on your mind. Once done, write about how you would like to feel instead, focusing on peace and forgiveness.
- **Breath Prayer:** Practice a simple breath prayer. Inhale deeply while saying, *"I release bitterness,"* and exhale while saying, *"I receive peace."* Repeat this for several minutes to center yourself.
- **Visualization:** Close your eyes and visualize a peaceful scene. Imagine letting go of your resentments, perhaps by visualizing them as leaves floating away on a stream. Allow yourself to feel the relief that comes with releasing those feelings.
- **Nightly Reflection:** Before bed, reflect on your day and write down any lingering feelings of resentment. Conclude with a prayer asking for God's help to release those feelings and embrace a restful night.
- **Calming Evening Ritual:** Establish a calming bedtime routine that includes reading Scripture, meditating on Ephesians 4:31, and spending a few moments in prayer for peace and forgiveness.

31 Days to Overcoming Insomnia

Write your responses here:

Day 30
EMBRACING FORGIVENESS

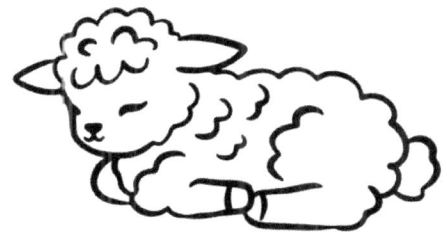

Romans 8:1 (KJV):
"There is therefore now no condemnation to them which are in Christ Jesus, who walk not after the flesh, but after the Spirit."

Imagine this: it is late at night, and everything outside is still. You pull back the blankets, you lie in your bed and shut your eyes, and you want to sleep. But then it happens. The conversation between the two of you starts coming back to you in your head from a few weeks before. A slight. A hurt. A word that was said, and a word that doesn't get out of your mouth anymore. You pull it back, but the thought keeps circling. Your heart races. Your muscles are tense. And then sleep is just another blurry memory.

Does this sound familiar? Unforgiveness is the thief who steals many people's quiet, sometimes during the night. It is the anger and the hurt, and it keeps us up in the night, going over the wrongs. It strips us of sleep when we're needing it most. Forgiveness, however, can break this cycle, liberating us from the attachment to the past and opening the door to true rest.

What if I told you that you are not only doing others an injustice, but you are also a key to your sleep, your health, and your harmony? But what if I told you there is no other thing in between you and the others you want?

No longer are you letting unforgiveness hold the reigns of your night, your day, and your life. Now let's discuss how forgiveness can make all the difference for you and how it can become the magic potion to getting better sleep.

The Cost of Holding On

Forgiveness is not about what happens when things get messy—it's about the way it affects our hearts, brains, and bodies. Forgiveness is a wallop, one that heaves us along and keeps us from going.

31 Days to Overcoming Insomnia

Consider all the times that you have been bitter or angry—at a friend, a family member, or even at yourself. You replay those episodes like a broken record in your head. The same cries of betrayal, hurt, and anger are felt again and again and each time they come to bite you just as much as when the offence occurred. It is not just your emotions that suffer from the weight of that anger; it's also your body that gets intruded and keeps you from getting rest. It makes you stressed, makes your muscles work harder and, above all, doesn't let you relax or sleep.

There is no rest if you have the emotional pain of old wounds. It's as if you are a person who is constantly with the world on their back and you don't know why you always feel drained, always bored. Until you're willing to forgive in the present moment, the hurt will stay with you, in waking life and when you're sleeping.

Romans 8:1 – The Word of God Is Free?
The reality is this: forgiveness is not an option—it is an obligation. It says in Romans 8:1 that *"There therefore is now no condemnation for those who are in Christ Jesus."* Let that sink in. No condemnation.

In Christ, you are not punished for what you have done wrong, nor are you punished for what other people have done. The slate is wiped clean. No more shame. No more guilt. And no longer should you feel any old hurts or offences. Forgive and you go out to live in this freedom.

The trouble is, forgiveness doesn't evince just to the other party. It's for you. It's for your peace. It's for you to be able to get on with life, to no longer let someone else's behavior determine your sleep and your life.

We will be saved in Christ because of Romans 8:1 where they promise that in Christ we are no longer condemned. That goes for the chastisement we give to ourselves and the chastisement of others. To forgive is to relinquish the ropes of guilt, rage, and resentment. You set free to exist in the peace Jesus died to redeem you from.

Forgiveness: The Pathway to Rest
Forgiveness is not an intellectual abstraction; it's all very real. It's the ticket to restorative sleep. Let me explain.

When you forgive, you no longer have to take over your life for those misdeeds from the past. You stop playing offence upon offence over and over, until they gain ever more grip over your brain. Rather, you decide in advance to give up, to let go of the rage, the hurt, and the bruise.

Unlock Deep Sleep Secrets

What happens when you forgive? Peace. Rest of heart, mind, and body. Forgiveness is where you throw your hurts down at the cross, and now your heart doesn't sink with all those hurts.

And the best part: after you get rid of that, you finally make room for rest and sleep. And no more do you take old problems with you in the night. Rather, you go to sleep knowing that you are not of this world. Forgiveness = rest.

Forgiveness is a Choice
You may be thinking: How can I forgive? It's hard when the suffering is so profound. But forgiveness is not a state of mind—it's an act.

1. Acknowledge the Hurt
Forgiveness starts with the hurt. You don't have to pretend the injury didn't happen. Face it. Feel it. Once you recognize the crime, then and only then, you can start to let it go.

2. Release the Desire for Revenge
Forgiveness often precedes an underlying wish for revenge or reparation. We wish to have the offending person "pay" for what he/she has done to us. But to forgive is to give up that wish. Forgiveness means you know that God will do it in His timing and the proper way. You let go of controlling the game.

3. Pray for the Power to Forgive
Forgiveness isn't always easy, and you may not be good at it. At those times, ask God for power. And then ask God to take the hurt and the resentment off of you and make your heart still. Keep in mind there is no condemnation for believers in Christ Jesus. He's forgiven you and by His grace, you can forgive people.

4. Choose Peace Over Pain
Forgiveness is about letting go rather than being hurt. There is no reversing the past, but you can respond to it. Forgive, and you are choosing forgiveness now, here, right now. You are refusing to be ruled by the past.

How Forgiveness Affects Your Sleep
Here is the bottom line: you can't sleep if you don't let go of your emotional baggage that's keeping you up at night. Forgiveness makes your head spin, your heart skip, and your muscles pound. Forgiveness removes you from all of that.

Imagine how much easier it will be when you decide to forgive. Now you'll stop feeling all that anger, bitterness, and grudges that were gnawing at your peace. You'll feel lighter and

31 Days to Overcoming Insomnia

freer. Your body will shut down, and your brain will slow down. And then you'll drift off into deep, peaceful sleep with the past at your back.

Sleep and Forgiveness — Two Powerful Tools in One
When you forgive, you aren't only repairing your relationships, but also your body, your mind, and your sleep. You don't just close your eyes at night to get sleep. It gives your body a place to rest, recharge, and heal. And you need silence to really sleep.

Forgiveness opens that door. That's the key to full mind, body, and soul reintegration. You deserve that rest. You want to go to sleep, a deep sleep, without having to feel that unforgiveness on your shoulders.

Prayer for the Journey
Dear God, thank you for the divine assurance given to me in Romans 1:8. It is so refreshing to know that I am free from condemnation because I am in Christ and I do not live out my life after the flesh but after the Spirit. This truth helps me resist the enemy's accusations about my past failures. Instead of rehearsing condemning thoughts, I choose to remind myself that I am forgiven, accepted, and covered by Your love. I rest in Your love, free from fear and guilt. I decree my sleep will be peaceful and secure in Your grace.

Help me to rest in the assurance of Your grace, and I decree that Your peace silences every accusing thought of the enemy. According to John 3:17, You did not send Your Son into the world to condemn the world, but that the world might be saved through Him. So, I release all anxiety now and I rest in the peace of Jesus. As I lay down to sleep tonight, my sleep will be sweet and my heart at rest, knowing that I am guiltless and secure in You. Amen.

Unlock Deep Sleep Secrets

JOURNAL
"Sound Sleep is Important"

Morning Cognitive Renewal Statements

- I release all guilt and embrace the freedom that comes from forgiveness. I am worthy of peace and rest.

Morning Journal Guided Reflections

Reflect on Guilt
Write about a specific situation or decision that causes you guilt. What feelings does this evoke? How does holding onto this guilt impact your day-to-day life?

_____
_____
_____

Setting Intentions
What is your intention for the day regarding letting go of guilt? Write down a specific action or mindset you wish to adopt.

_____
_____
_____
_____

Gratitude Practice
List three things you are grateful for this morning. Reflect on how focusing on gratitude can help shift your attention away from guilt.

- I am grateful for _____
- I am thankful for _____
- I appreciate for _____

Self-Compassion Reflection
Think about an area where you struggle to forgive yourself. What is one kind thing you can say to yourself today to promote self-compassion?

_____
_____
_____
_____

31 Days to Overcoming Insomnia

Afternoon Journal Guided Reflections

Midday Check-In
Reflect on your day so far. Have any feelings of guilt surfaced? Write about how you handled these emotions and what you learned from them.

_____
_____
_____
_____
_____
_____
_____

Forgiveness Letter
Write a letter to yourself expressing forgiveness for past mistakes. Acknowledge your feelings and remind yourself that it's okay to let go.

_____
_____
_____
_____
_____
_____
_____

Prayer for Release
Spend a few moments in prayer, asking God to help you release guilt and embrace His forgiveness. Be specific about what you want to let go of.

Supportive Connection
Share your journey with a trusted friend or family member. Discuss how guilt affects your emotional state and seek their perspective on forgiveness.

Evening Mindful Rest Practices

- **Guilt-Release Meditation**
  Engage in a guided meditation focused on releasing guilt. Visualize the burdens you carry and imagine them dissipating as you breathe deeply, inviting peace into your heart.

- **Journaling Exercise**
  Create a page titled "Letting Go of Guilt." Write down specific instances of guilt you wish to release. Afterward, consider a symbolic act, like tearing up the page or burning it, to signify your release.

Unlock Deep Sleep Secrets

- **Mindfulness Breathing**
  Practice a breathing exercise: Inhale deeply while saying, "I am free," and exhale while saying, "I let go of guilt." Repeat this for several minutes, focusing on the sensations of relief and calm.

- **Calming Evening Routine**
  Establish a soothing bedtime ritual that includes reading Romans 8:1, reflecting on your day, and meditating on the idea of release. Spend time in prayer, asking for peace and comfort as you prepare for sleep.

- **Creative Expression**
  Create a piece of art that represents your journey of letting go of guilt. Use colors, images, and words that resonate with feelings of release, healing, and freedom.

Day 31
SILENT MIND, RESTFUL SLEEP: NAVIGATING YOUR SUBCONSCIOUS

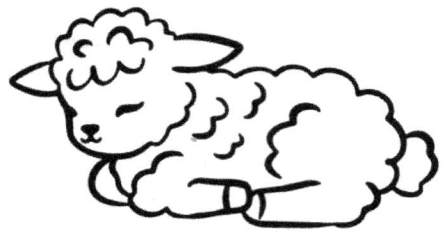

Matthew 6:22-23 (KJV):
"The light of the body is the eye: if therefore thine eye be single, thy whole body shall be full of light. But if thine eye be evil, thy whole body."

Matthew 6:22-23 – The Eye is the Lamp of the Body

But if you want to know how to work with your subconscious mind in sleep, let's begin with this amazing passage from Matthew 6:22-23: *'The eye is the lamp of the body. You'll be bright all the time if your eyes are okay. But your body is dark all the time, if your eyes are bad. If then that darkness in which you are dwelling is darkness, how great is that darkness!'*

These verses appear on the surface to be about the eye. But on a more fundamental level, they're talking about how we perceive the external world—and how that perception is what shapes our inner world, including our subconscious. It's our brains that are like mirrors with which we judge all the things that we see, hear, and experience. What we pay attention to, what we put in our brain, becomes "the light" or "darkness" in us.

The energy that you allow to come into your mind through negativity, stress, and buried emotions will be stored by your subconscious mind and stored in the form of "darkness" that can mess up your sleep. But if you decide to focus on quietness, joy, good thoughts, you send the light in. And that light plays havoc with your waking and subconscious, with how you sleep, and how well you get to sleep.

Consider this: your subconscious mind is a sponge that receives everything you get from the day. You just clutter it up with so much stress and that is what it will be like at night when

Unlock Deep Sleep Secrets

you're sleeping. But if you decorate it with light (good things), by meditating and getting rid of the stresses of the day, it will always feel like an ideal space for sleeping.

The Mind and the Mind-Power of Ideas

Your subconscious brain is just that good. It does almost everything on autopilot—from breathing to your reaction to stress. Indeed, most of our daily behaviors, thoughts, and emotions are probably dictated by the subconscious. And this is the secret to sleep harmony.

And here's the catch: the subconscious does not speak like the conscious. It thinks in pictures, sensations, and feelings. It retorts to the same thoughts and beliefs—for better or worse. The more you focus on something, either in conscious or subconscious form, the more that thought stays with you in your unconscious mind and impacts your emotional and mental well-being.

Your subconscious Is not just stuc" on 'tress, anxiety, or unmet needs; it's just stuck on the pattern—which is much harder to shut off in the evenings. It all starts with learning how powerful your thoughts are, and deliberately redirecting them in a direction of relaxation, tranquility, and rest.

The Role of Focus in Your Sleep

And Matthew 6:22-23 connects the focus to which we have given complete attention to the state of mind and body in general. If we think about light, peace, thanksgiving, and positive thoughts, all of our bodies and minds are filled with the peace. But if we dwell on the dark—on unfinished business, anxieties, and self-doubts—we will take that burden with us into bed.

When it comes to sleep, that is, what you are paying attention to just before you close your eyes matters. Your subconscious is most susceptible to the morning before you go to bed. If you go to bed still writhing in your brain because you're stressed, anxious, or angry, you are letting those emotions get in your subconscious mind, where they will hang around, disrupting your sleep. But if you train it to be peaceful, quiet, and grateful, then you're "training" your unconscious to sleep.

Prayer for the Journey

Dear God, this evening's entry will be the last in my journal; therefore, I thank you for the progress I've made through these 31 days. Thank you for Your word that reminds me of the importance of where to fix my eyes both spiritually and mentally. If I allow my mind to be consumed with worry, fear, greed, or sinful distractions, then I will be filled with restlessness, anxiety, and despair. But if I keep my eyes on Your goodness and Your truth, my life will be filled with light peace, joy, and clarity.

I struggle with sleepless nights due to racing thoughts, negative influences, and stress. Help me not to allow fear, bitterness, or worldly concerns to dominate my mind, but show

31 Days to Overcoming Insomnia

me how to shift my focus on Your word – Your promises and Your love- which lead to peace and rest.

I decree that my spiritual eyes are single, focused only on You. Lord let Your light fill my heart; bring clarity where there is confusion, peace where there is anxiety, and rest where there is restlessness. Let my sleep be sweet, undisturbed by the worries of this world. I declare that my mind is fixed on You; consequently, I will rest in perfect peace. Your peace will become the guiding force in my subconscious mind during the night as it leads me with clarity and serenity.

Thank you for being the light of my salvation. Thank you for keeping me in perfect peace because my mind is stayed on You. Your word is a lamp unto my feet and a path to find perfect rest; therefore, I will rest in Your presence tonight in Jesus' name. Amen.

Unlock Deep Sleep Secrets

JOURNAL
"Sound Sleep is Important"

Morning Cognitive Renewal Statements

- I choose to see with clarity and focus on thoughts that bring light and positivity into my life. My mind is a source of peace and strength.

Morning Journal Guided Reflections

Intention for the Day: What positive intention can I set today to guide my thoughts and actions? How can I keep my focus on the light?

_____
_____
_____
_____

Self-Discovery: What qualities or strengths do I want to embrace today? How can I express them in my interactions?

_____
_____
_____
_____
_____
_____
_____
_____

Positive Visualization: Visualize how I want my day to unfold. What feelings do I want to carry with me throughout the day?

_____
_____
_____
_____
_____
_____
_____
_____

Evening Journal Guided Reflections

31 Days to Overcoming Insomnia

Gratitude Reflection: What three things am I grateful for today? How did they bring light into my day?

- I am grateful for _____
- I am thankful for _____
- I appreciate for _____

What I am grateful for will bring light by:
_____
_____
_____
_____
_____

What I am thankful for will bring light by:
_____
_____
_____
_____
_____

What I am thankful for will bring light by:
_____
_____
_____
_____
_____

Thought Inventory
Did I encounter any negative or unhelpful thoughts today? What were those thoughts? How can I reframe them into something positive and constructive?
_____
_____
_____
_____
_____
_____
_____

Unlock Deep Sleep Secrets

Subconscious Insights
Before sleep, write down any dreams or lingering thoughts. What insights do they provide about my inner self?

_____
_____
_____
_____
_____
_____
_____
_____
_____
_____
_____

Evening Mindful Rest Practices

- **Mindful Meditation**
  Dedicate 5-10 minutes each morning to meditate. Focus on your breath and visualize light filling your mind. Ask yourself, "What do I need to see clearly today?"

- **Journaling**
  Keep a dedicated journal for exploring your subconscious. Spend 10-15 minutes writing freely about your thoughts and feelings. Afterward, review what you've written to identify patterns or themes.

- **Affirmation Practice**
  Create a list of affirmations that resonate with you. Repeat them each morning to reinforce positive beliefs and clarity. Examples include: *"I am worthy of love and peace,"* or *"I see the light in every situation."*

- **Nature Connection**
  Spend time outdoors, observing how natural light changes your perception. Reflect on how being in nature can help clear your mind and connect you to your inner thoughts.

- **Visualization Exercise**
  Before sleep, visualize a scenario where you are free from negativity. Picture yourself surrounded by light and positivity, allowing that image to guide you into a peaceful sleep.

- **Scripture Reflection**

31 Days to Overcoming Insomnia

Spend time meditating on Matthew 6:22-23. Reflect on how your perceptions shape your inner thoughts. Write down any insights you gain and how they can influence your day.

- **Final Thoughts**
By incorporating these prompts, affirmations, and activities into your sound sleep journal, you can create a meaningful practice that promotes self-awareness and clarity. This exploration will not only enhance your understanding of your subconscious, but it will also support you in cultivating a peaceful and restful sleep.

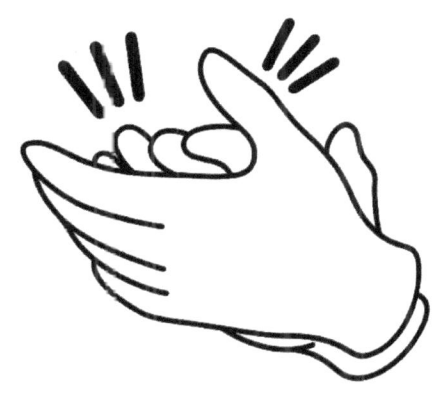

**WAY TO GO!!!
YOU HAVE COMPLETED
YOUR 31-DAY JOURNEY!**

Conclusion
MOVING FORWARD IN CONTINUOUS SOUND SLEEP AND REJUVENATION

You did it. You finished a staggering 31-day journey but you shouldn't relax yet. This isn't the end. Oh no. It's the beginning of something huge. The sleep you've unlocked is only a preview of the power you now control. Picture yourself maximizing every piece of knowledge you've gathered by pushing it to its ultimate intensity. Take advantage of your recent progress to catapult yourself into a lifestyle far exceeding your wildest dreams.

Are you prepared to plunge into a future where you maintain constant energy levels combined with intense focus and wake up daily feeling completely refreshed? You stand at the brink of entering an entirely fresh reality. And the best part? This isn't a one-time fix—it's a lifestyle.

What's Next? The Future You Didn't Know You Could Have
Look at where you are now. You've already begun the transformation. Remember how you started this journey? Exhausted, frustrated, struggling through sleepless nights? That version of you is gone. You have invested time into changing your sleep patterns and now wake up each day feeling more alert and purposeful.

Take It Further—The Next Level of Sleep Mastery
You've learned the basics, but now it's time to push yourself beyond what you thought was possible. The strategies you've put into practice are *working*. But imagine how much more powerful your life will become when you take it to the next level.

Here's how to do it:

1. **Make Sleep Your Superpower:** This goes beyond simply going to sleep and waking up. This is about making sleep the foundation of your life. You have the opportunity to rejuvenate your mind, spirit, and body every night. Consider making bedtime a sacred ritual, a time to strengthen your most important resource: yourself. Sleep turns into your secret weapon when you intentionally go through this process.

2. **Adapt Like a Sleep Ninja:** You will face obstacles in life. It always does. But now? You're prepared. Regardless of what life throws at you, you will face obstacles in life. Stressful day, your sleep won't suffer. Unforeseen events? our sleep will always be

Unlock Deep Sleep Secrets

revered. Nothing can topple the system you've established. And you'll overcome every challenge with that strength.

3. **Track Your Growth—And Push Your Limits:** You started tracking your sleep for a meaningful purpose. But that's just the beginning. You possess the ability to understand how sleep influences every aspect of your life including your mood and energy levels together with your creativity and decision-making abilities. Want to go deeper? Track your dreams, your emotions, your productivity. By monitoring both your sleep patterns and energy fluctuations you gain valuable knowledge which enables you to make precise adjustments that enhance your life beyond your expectations. You're just scratching the surface.

4. **Master Your Mindset—Sleep is the Key:** The power of sleep to transform your body has been demonstrated, so it's time to explore its effects on your mind. Sleep patterns directly influence your mental framework by determining your thoughts and beliefs which together construct your entire life. Correct sleep optimization leads your mind to achieve sharper thinking abilities, quicker problem-solving skills and extended focus periods. So, what's next? Picture a mind that always maintains clarity and sharpness to address any challenge. Sleep acts as your mental reset button while you continue to hold the key.

5. **Celebrate Every Win—You've Earned It:** The tendency to ignore small victories existed until now. Achieving a good night's sleep represents a significant achievement. When you wake up each day filled with energy and clarity while feeling motivated you take a significant step in your journey forward. This transformation means more than just completing tasks because it focuses on acknowledging your journey and valuing all steps of progress. Every small victory deserves celebration because when combined they create significant achievements.

Final Activation: Unlock Your Limitless Future

This is where magic happens. You've already felt the change. You've already witnessed what's possible. But now, we're going to lock it in. We're going to turn the power you've just unlocked into something *unstoppable*.

Step 1: Reflect on Your Journey—The Power Is Yours
Look back. Focus on your transformation rather than your struggle. You've evolved from battling sleepless nights to starting your days full of energy and prepared to face everything. Let that sink in. This is real. This is happening.

31 Days to Overcoming Insomnia

Step 2: Visualize Your Ultimate Sleep
Envision the amazing sensation of having legendary sleep instead of just good sleep. Experience mental sharpness paired with powerful energy flowing through your body every morning when you wake up completely rejuvenated each day. When you utilize sleep to empower your life you can achieve every dream you've ever imagined.

Step 3: Write Your Declaration of Power
It's time to make it official. Write it down: "I am the master of my sleep. I choose to thrive, not just survive. Each night I fall into deep sleep and every new day starts with me feeling energized and focused to build my ideal life. Write it. Believe it. Make this promise your personal commitment to yourself.

Step 4: Activate Tonight
Don't wait for tomorrow. Start tonight. Make your sleep routine a sacred ritual. Create a plan for a restful night that revitalizes you so you can face the next day with energy and determination.

Conclusion: This Is Just the Beginning
The greatest resource to enhance your life has just been revealed to you through sleep. This marks not the conclusion of your journey but rather the start of a new chapter in your life. Through every night of restful sleep and every morning of renewed energy and mental clarity you continue to evolve into your amazing, destined self.

This is your time. This is your moment.

If you're prepared to move forward, you'll become unstoppable as you ascend to new heights—watch out world.

Go. Unleash your potential. You've got this.